Fundamentals of ETHICS AND GOOD CLINICAL PRACTICE IN RESEARCH

Chief Editors:

Dr. Anupma Jyoti Kindo

Dr. Swati Kumari

Dr. Linga Devi T

notionpress.com

INDIA • SINGAPORE • MALAYSIA

ISBN
Paperback 979-8-90362-936-7
Hardcase 979-8-90431-267-1

SRI RAMACHANDRA

INSTITUTE OF HIGHER EDUCATION AND RESEARCH

(Deemed to be University)

Dr. MAHESH VAKAMUDI, MD (Anaesthesiology)
PRO VICE-CHANCELLOR

Porur, Chennai - 600 116
Phone : 091-44-2476 5625
Email : provc@sriramachandra.edu.in
www.sriramachandra.edu.in

FOREWORD

Ethics is the cornerstone of scientific inquiry, especially in research involving human participants. In an era of rapid technological innovation and the globalization of clinical trials, adherence to Good Clinical Practice (GCP) and robust ethical standards is not merely a regulatory requirement but a moral imperative.

I am pleased to introduce *Fundamentals of Good Clinical Practice and Research Ethics*, a timely and essential contribution to academic and professional training. Developed in alignment with University Grants Commission (UGC) and Indian Council of Medical Research (ICMR) guidelines, this work reflects a deep commitment to scientific integrity and ethical rigor.

What distinguishes this textbook is the expertise of its authors. The chapters are penned by seasoned members of Institutional Ethics Committees from Sri Ramachandra Institute of Higher Education and Research (SRIHER). Their extensive experience in ethical review and regulatory oversight lends the text a practical authority that goes beyond pure theory.

The book comprehensively covers the essential aspects of research ethics, including respect for persons, beneficence, justice, and informed consent—while addressing modern challenges in digital health, artificial intelligence, and multicentric trials. This forward-looking approach ensures readers are well-equipped for the evolving research landscape.

Whether you are a postgraduate student, a clinical investigator, or an ethics committee professional, this textbook is an invaluable resource. I commend the editors and contributors for their dedication to advancing these standards. I highly recommend it to everyone committed to excellence and integrity in clinical research.

PRO VICE-CHANCELLOR

Chief Editor's Note

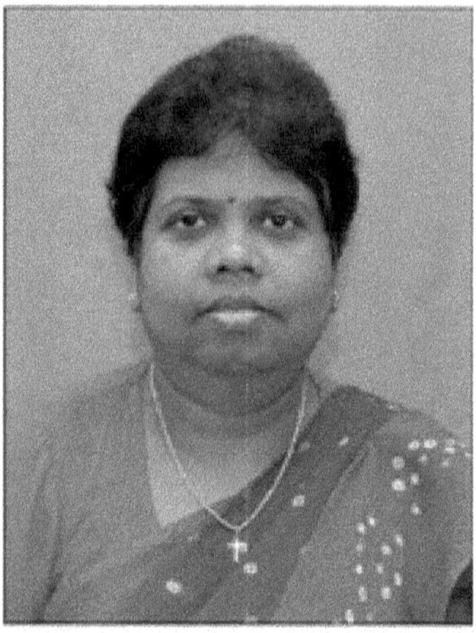

It gives me immense pleasure to present this scholarly work on *Fundamentals of Ethics and Good Clinical Practice in Research*, authored by the experienced and expert members of the Institutional Ethics Committee of Sri Ramachandra Institute of Higher Education and Research (SRIHER). This book would have not been possible without the support and unwavering guidance of our Pro Vice Chancellor Dr.Mahesh Vakamudi whose constant encouragement has been instrumental in shaping this book from its conception to completion.

In this contemporary era of scientific advancement and ethical integrity strict adherence to Good Clinical Practice serves as an indispensable pillar of responsible research. With increasing emphasis on transparency, participant safety, and regulatory compliance, it becomes imperative for research scholars to possess a sound understanding of ethical principles and guidelines governing clinical and biomedical research.

This book is a timely and valuable contribution, particularly for PhD scholars, as it comprehensively addresses the core concepts of research ethics, regulatory frameworks, informed consent, safety reporting, and ethical review processes. It aligns well with the requirements of research methodology training as prescribed by the University Grants Commission (UGC), making it an essential resource for scholars preparing for their doctoral examinations. The strength of this book is in its practical orientation, clarity of concepts, and relevance to real-world research scenarios. The collective expertise of the authors, drawn from their extensive experience in ethics committee functioning, ensures that the content is both authoritative and applicable. I sincerely acknowledge all the authors and institutional support that made this book possible. I am hopeful that this book will serve as a guiding tool for research scholars, faculty members, and healthcare professionals, fostering a culture of ethical research and scientific excellence.

Dr. Anupma Jyoti Kindo

Professor (former Head) Department of Microbiology

Member Secretary of IEC , SRIHER

Acknowledgement

We extend our sincere gratitude to Pro Vice Chancellor, SRIHER, Dr. Mahesh Vakamudi, for his continued encouragement, guidance, and institutional support, which have been instrumental in the successful completion of this book titled " *Fundamentals of Ethics and Good Clinical Practice in Research* ".

This book, would not have been possible without the steadfast support and inspiring guidance of Dr. Anupma Jyoti Kindo, Chief editor whose constant encouragement, academic leadership, and commitment to excellence have been a source of inspiration throughout the development of this work. Her dedicated and committed approach, coupled with her compassionate and motherly guidance, has profoundly influenced and motivated us at every stage of this endeavour. Her emphasis on ethical standards, quality research, and academic integrity has indeed significantly shaped the content and direction of this book.

We extend our deepest appreciation to all the esteemed authors —members of the Ethics Committee and subject experts—whose vast experience and dedication have enriched this book. Their commitment to advancing knowledge in research ethics and good clinical practice has been invaluable. We also acknowledge the support of our institution SRIHER and all staff and secretarial assistance who have directly or indirectly contributed to the successful completion of this book.

This book, from its conception to publication, has taken us on a remarkable journey—one that not only enriched our knowledge but also brought us closer together, strengthening our bond as part of the SRIHER family. The countless hours, endless discussions, and shared good humor have carried us forward and made this journey truly memorable.

Finally we would like to extend thanks to our families for their unwavering love, patience, and understanding throughout this journey. Their constant moral support and love provided the strength and motivation needed to bring this work to completion.

We are sure that students, researchers, and healthcare professionals will enjoy reading and greatly benefit from the information provided in this book.

Dr. Swati Kumari

Dr. Lingadevi Thanasekaran

Chief Editors

Author's Write-up

This book serves as a comprehensive guide for PhD scholars for their UGC based paper on research and publication ethics and faculty members navigating the complex landscape of medical research and publication ethics. It is specifically designed to bridge the gap between theoretical ethical principles and their practical application in clinical trials and academic writing.

The content is aligned with the latest national and international regulatory frameworks. It covers the essential-ICMR National Ethical and AI Guidelines for biomedical research, the CDSCO New Drugs and Clinical Trials Rules and GCP guidelines.

Readers will find practical explanations of standards and guidelines, ensuring that research data is credible and participant rights are protected. A significant portion of the book is dedicated to research ethics, publications ethics addressing critical issues like authorship criteria, conflict of interest, and the prevention of misconduct such as plagiarism and data fabrication.

By simplifying rigorous guidelines into actionable steps, this book empowers researchers to conduct high-quality, ethical studies that meet global standards. It is an indispensable resource for anyone committed to maintaining the integrity and sanctity of medical science and ethical and responsible conduct of the research. It is easy to understand and also very useful for exam preparation for PhD scholars for paper on research and publication ethics.

Quote-Neil Armstrong's famous first words upon stepping on the moon was : "That's one small step for [a] man, one giant leap for mankind". The authors believe this book is the first step towards having an army of ethical and responsible researchers.

Happy ethical responsible research learning for years to come!

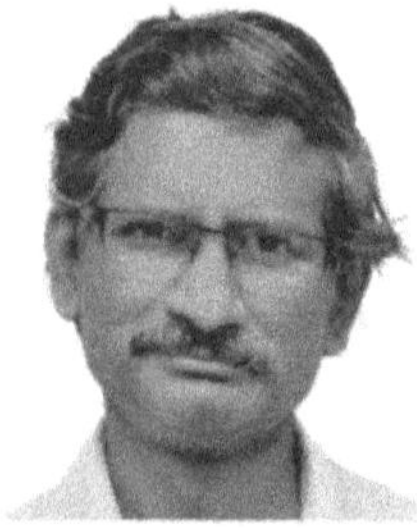

Dr Emmanuel Bhaskar
Professor, Department of Medicine
SRIHER
IEC Member 9 years and member secretary
Email: drebhaskar@ sriramachandra.edu.in
9840717971

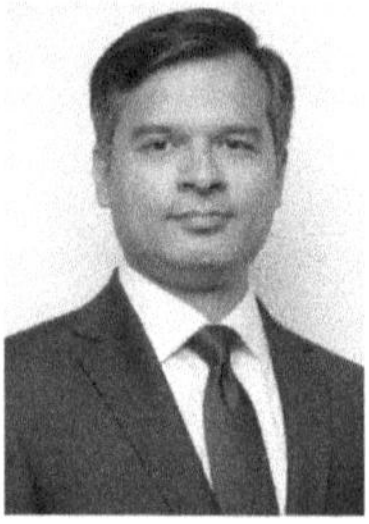

Dr. Rajesh Kumar Gandhirajan,
Professor, Department of Human Genetics
Faculty of Biomedical Sciences and Technology
SRIHER
Mobile: 7200245971
Email: rajesh.gandhirajan@ sriramachandra.edu.in

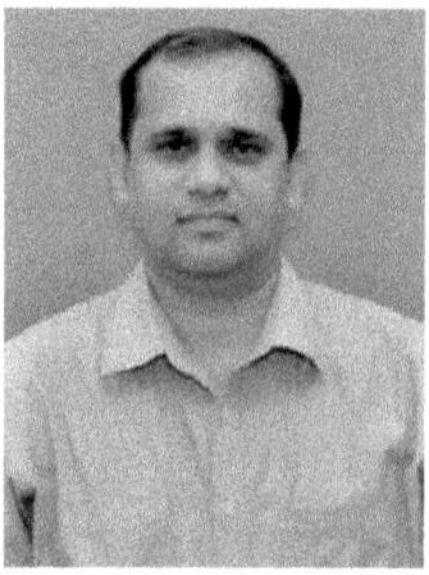

Dr. Pankaj B.Shah
Associate Dean Research, Professor, Former Professor & Head dept of Community Medicine,SRIHER,
IEC Experience for 15 years
drpankajbshah@gmail.com
pankajbshah@ sriramachandra.edu.in

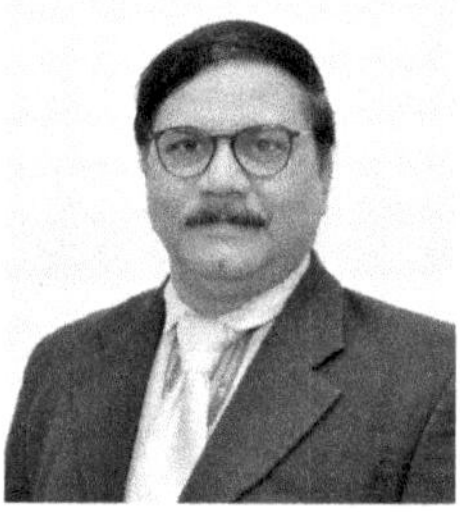

Dr. Krishnendu Mukhopadhyay
Professor, EHE,Faculty of Public Health,SRIHER
Teaching experience 25 years and Research experience 30 years.IEC experience about 10 years.
kmjalika1967@gmail.com;/ krishnendu@ sriramachandra.edu.in

<table>
<tr>
<td>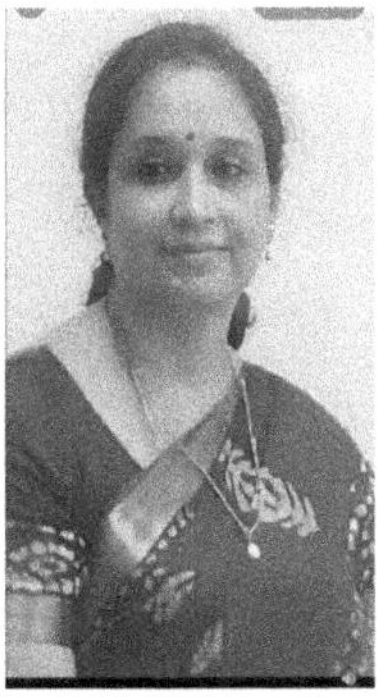
Dr.D.Anusha
Professor,Department of pharmacology,SRIHER
Teaching experience 19 years ,IEC experience 12 years since 2014
E Mail: drdanusha@gmail.com / anusha.d@sriramachandra.edu.in</td>
<td>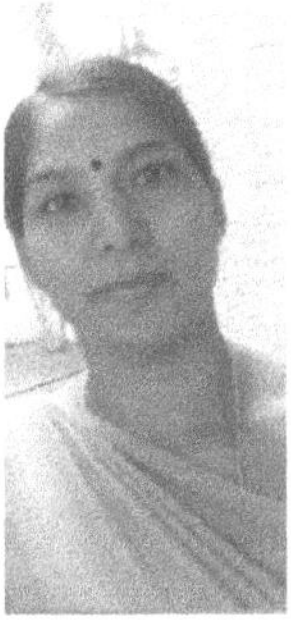
Dr. T. Gayathri
Assistant Professor,Dept of Community Medicine,SRIHER
IEC Experience - 10 years, teaching experience 25 years
gayathristat19@gmail/ gayathri.t@ sriramachandra.edu.in</td>
</tr>
<tr>
<td>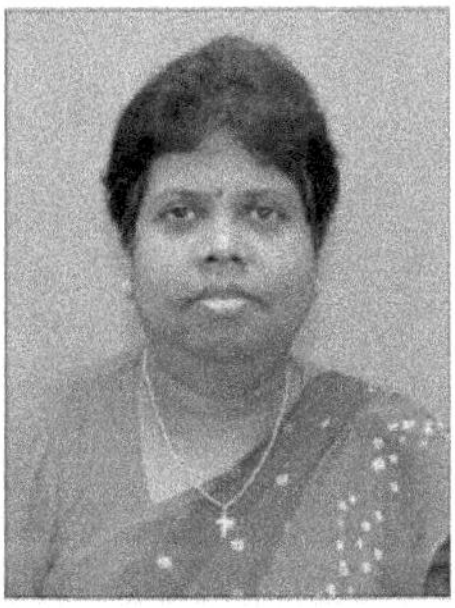
Dr.Anupma Kindo
Professor (former head department of Microbiology), SRIHER
Member secretary of IEC , 10 years as member of IEC,28 years of teaching experience
anupmalakra@gmail.com / anupamajyoti@ sriramachandra.edu.in</td>
<td>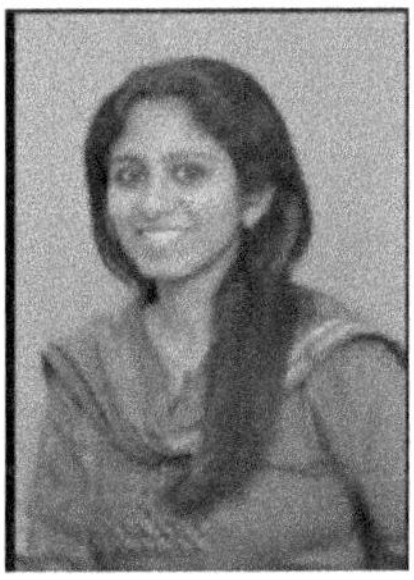
Dr.Linga devi Thanasekaran
Coordinator of Centre for Professional Development , SRIHER
Teaching Experience 15 years in UK and India .Institutional ethics committee member of SRIHER for 7 years for both Undergraduate and postgraduate students at SRIHER.
drlinga2@gmail.com /lingadevi@ sriramachandra.edu.in</td>
</tr>
</table>

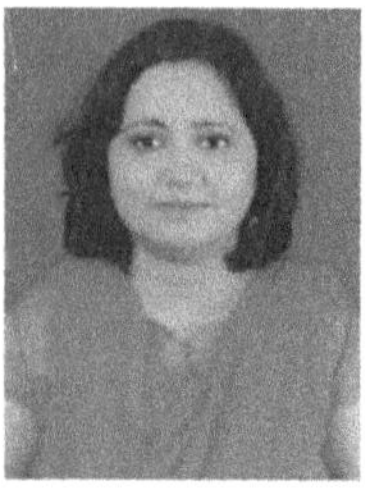

Dr. Swati Kumari
Assistant Professor,Department of Microbiology,SRIHER
Teaching Experience: 10 years and Research Experience: 6 years
IEC Experience as senior member of postgraduate ethics committee for 6 months
Email drswatikumari@sriramachandra.edu.in/drswatimicro@gmail.com

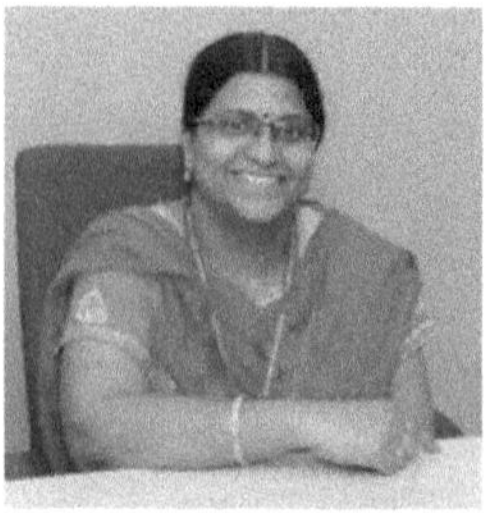

Dr. T.Mohanapriya
Professor, General Surgery,SRIHER
Teaching experience 18 years and Research experience 15 years.
IEC experience about 7 years.
mohanapriyadr@gmail.com;mohanapriyadr@sriramachandra.edu.in

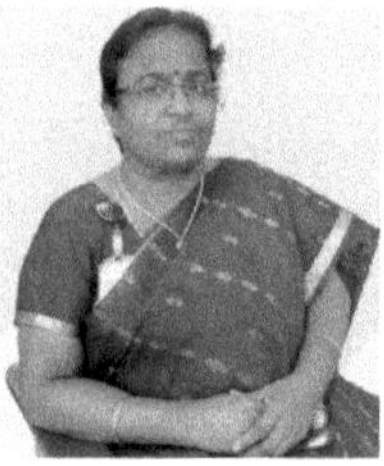

Dr. Aruna Subramaniam
Professor and HOD-Sri Ramachandra Faculty of Nursing,SRIHER
26 years of teaching experience, 8 years of iec experience as member secretary 5 years
Mail id : aruna.s@sriramachandra.edu.in/arunga666666@gmail.com

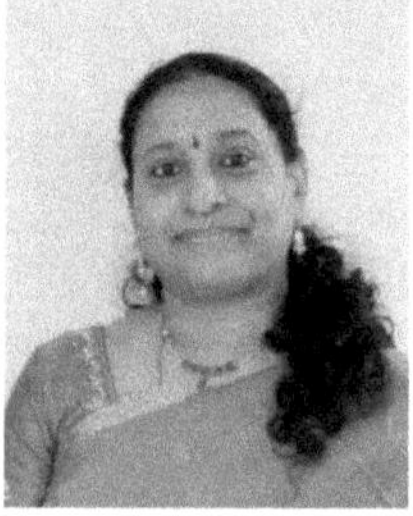

Dr.Divyambika CV
Professor,Department of Oral Medicine and Radiology ,SRIHER
Teaching experience -18 years,IEC experience - 3 years,IEC Member Secretary since 2 years
cvdivyambika@sriramachandra.edu.in /drdivyambika@gmail.com

Contents

Chief Editor's Note *4*

Acknowledgement *6*

Author's Write-up *8*

1. Philosophy and Ethical Guidelines in India 15
2. Scientific Conduct and Research Misconduct 44
3. Publication Ethics in Research: Plagiarism, Predatory Journals and Predatory Conferences 61
4. Open Access Publishing and Ethics in Digital Research 91
5. Publication Misconduct 119
6. Databases and Research Metrics 145
7. Composition and Functions of Institutional Ethics Committees 166
8. Good Clinical Practice and Clinical Trial 211
9. Ethical Issues in Study Designs and Statistics 256
10. Informed Consent 267
11. Serious Adverse Drug Events (SAEs) And Ethical Reporting 282
12. Data Protection and Privacy in Research-Ethics 309

Annexure 1 *329*

Annexure 2 *332*

Synopsis *334*

Chapter1

Philosophy and Ethical Guidelines in India

Dr.Pankaj B. Shah
Associate Dean Research, Professor
Department of Community Medicine
pankajbshah@gmail.com

Abstract:

This chapter outlines key international and national guidelines governing human research ethics, including ICMR and ICH-GCP. It highlights core ethical principles, informed consent, confidentiality, risk–benefit assessment, and protection of vulnerable populations, along with emerging issues such as AI and regulatory frameworks in India.

Keywords:

Research Ethics; ICMR; ICH-GCP; Informed Consent; Confidentiality; Clinical Trials; Regulatory Framework

Objectives:

- List important guidelines and laws for research ethics in International and National context
- Describe salient features of important guidelines and laws for research ethics in International and National context

Introduction:

Ethics means doing what is right. Medical ethics has a long history in India. Ancient texts like Charaka Samhita spoke about "do no harm". Research helps to improve health. It increases knowledge about diseases. It develops new medicines and treatments. But research can also cause harm. Participants may face physical, mental, social or financial risks. Therefore, ethical guidelines are necessary.

Clinical research and healthcare innovation are growing rapidly in India and globally. New medicines, vaccines, medical devices and artificial intelligence tools are being developed every year. These developments bring hope for better treatment and improved patient care. At the same time, they also bring responsibility. Research involving human participants must follow ethical standards. Regulatory processes must ensure safety and transparency. Digital systems must protect data privacy and security.

International and national guidelines guide this entire ecosystem. The International Council for Harmonisation Good Clinical Practice guideline provides global standards for clinical trials. The Indian Council of Medical Research provides ethical guidance for biomedical research and artificial intelligence in healthcare. The Central Drugs Standard Control Organisation regulates drugs and medical devices in India and provides the SUGAM portal for online regulatory submissions.

All these frameworks together form a strong system. This system protects research participants. It ensures scientific validity. It builds public trust. It promotes innovation while safeguarding rights and safety.

Indian Council of Medical Research ethical guidelines:

The Indian Council of Medical Research (ICMR) provides ethical guidance for biomedical and health research in India. These guidelines apply to academic institutions, hospitals and industry-sponsored research.

Ethical Foundations:

- The guidelines are based on respect for persons, beneficence and justice. Respect means autonomy. Participants have the right to decide. Beneficence means do good and avoid harm. Justice means fair selection of participants.
- Vulnerable populations need special protection. These include children, pregnant women, economically disadvantaged persons and people with limited literacy.
- Informed consent must be clear and understandable. Confidentiality must be maintained. Compensation for research-related injury must be provided.
- Ethics Committees must be registered and follow standard operating procedures
- All research, including conference presentations, should be approved by the ethics committee before the start of the study.
- Clinical trial registration is mandatory for all experimental studies, including clinical trials.

Biomedical and health research plays an important role in improving healthcare in India. It helps develop new medicines, new treatments, and better public health policies. Hence, research involving human participants must be conducted carefully. Human beings have dignity. They have rights. Their safety and well-being must always be protected. The Indian Council of Medical Research released ethical guidelines in 1980. These were revised in 2000 and 2006. The latest version came out in 2017.

To guide researchers in India, the Indian Council of Medical Research released the National Ethical Guidelines for Biomedical and Health Research Involving Human Participants in 2017. These guidelines provide a strong ethical framework for all types of research involving humans.

The guidelines apply to clinical trials, public health research, social and behavioural research, genetics research, and research involving biological samples or data. They apply to government institutions, private hospitals, universities and industry-sponsored studies. The purpose of the guidelines is to ensure that research is scientifically valid and ethically sound. Ethical research builds trust between researchers and society. Without trust, research cannot progress.

The foundation of these guidelines is based on certain core ethical principles. The first principle is respect for persons. Every participant must be treated with dignity. Individuals have the right to make their own decisions. They should not be forced or misled into participating in research. Respect also means protecting privacy and maintaining confidentiality. The second principle is beneficence. Research should aim to benefit participants or society. It should contribute to better knowledge or improved healthcare. The third principle is non-maleficence. This means that researchers must avoid causing harm. Even if research has potential benefits, unnecessary risks must not be taken. The fourth principle is justice. The burdens and benefits of research must be shared fairly. No group should be unfairly burdened or excluded without reason.

Before starting any research, the risks and benefits must be carefully assessed. Research should begin only if the potential benefits justify the risks involved. If the risks are too high and the expected benefit is small, the research should not proceed. Risk assessment is not a one-time activity. It must continue throughout the study. If new risks arise, they must be addressed immediately. Participants must be informed about any new information that may affect their willingness to continue.

One of the most important parts of ethical research is the process of informed consent. Informed consent is not just a signature on a paper. It is a continuous process of communication between the researcher and the participant. Participants must be given complete and understandable information about the purpose of the research, the procedures involved, the risks and possible benefits, and their right to withdraw at any time. The language used must be simple. Technical terms should be avoided. Participants must be given enough time to think and ask questions. Consent must be voluntary. There should be no pressure, threat or undue influence or inducement.

Special care must be taken when participants are illiterate or have limited understanding. In such cases, the consent form must be explained clearly in the local language. An impartial witness may be required. Audio-visual recording of the consent process may be used in some types of studies as per regulatory guidelines.

Privacy and confidentiality are essential elements of research ethics. Participants share personal health information. They may also share sensitive social or genetic information. This information must be protected. Data should be stored securely. Access must be restricted. Identifiable information should not be disclosed without permission. When data is published, it should not reveal the identity of participants. Protecting confidentiality builds confidence and encourages participation in research.

Some individuals and groups are vulnerable. Vulnerability may arise due to age, illness, disability, economic condition, or social disadvantage. Children, pregnant women, tribal communities, prisoners and persons with mental illness are considered vulnerable groups. Research involving such groups requires additional safeguards. Inclusion of vulnerable groups must be scientifically justified. Researchers must ensure that these groups are not exploited. For children, parental consent is required along with assent from the child, depending on age and maturity (till 7 years, parental consent; 7-12 years, oral assent in addition to parental consent; 12-18 years, written assent in addition to parental consent).

Ethical principles:

A. There are four core principles:

1. Respect for persons
2. Beneficence
3. Non-maleficence
4. Justice

B. These are expanded into 12 general principles:

1. Essentiality
2. Voluntariness

3. Non-exploitation
4. Social Responsibility
5. Privacy and Confidentiality
6. Risk Minimisation
7. Professional Competence
8. Maximisation of Benefit
9. Institutional Arrangements
10. Transparency and Accountability
11. Total Responsibility
12. Environmental Protection

C. The key ethical concerns:

1. Benefit-Risk Assessment:

Benefits must outweigh risks.

Risks can be physical, mental, social or economic.

Risk categories:

- Less than minimal risk
- Minimal risk
- Minor increase over minimal risk
- More than minimal risk

Ethics Committees assess risk before approval.

2. Informed Consent:

Informed consent protects autonomy.

It has three parts:

- Information
- Understanding
- Voluntary agreement

Consent must be:

- In simple language
- In local language
- Signed and documented

If participant cannot consent, Legal Authorised Representative gives consent.

3. Privacy and Confidentiality:

Personal data must be protected.

Sensitive data such as HIV status or genetic information must be handled with care. Additionally, separate guidelines for HIV and genetics should be followed.

4. Distributive Justice:

Benefits and burdens must be shared fairly.

Vulnerable groups must not be exploited.

5. Payment for Participation:

Participants may receive:

- Travel reimbursement.
- Compensation for time.

But payment must not become an undue inducement.

6. Compensation for Research-Related Harm:

If harm occurs:

- Free medical care must be given.
- Compensation must be provided.

Serious Adverse Events must be reported as per the latest guidelines.

7. Conflict of Interest:

8. Community Engagement:

9. Post-Research Access:

Participants should benefit after the study ends.

Access to drugs or services should be planned in advance.

D. Responsible Conduct of Research:

Responsible research builds public trust.

Core Values:

- Honesty
- Accuracy
- Accountability
- Transparency

Mentoring:

Senior researchers must guide juniors. Ethical behaviour must be taught.

Policies:

Institutions must:

- Protect participants
- Have research offices
- Provide training
- Monitor research

Animal Research:

Must follow national laws and humane guidelines.

Data Management:

Data must be:

- Properly recorded
- Safely stored
- Backed up, archival as per guidelines
- Shared responsibly

Participants own their biological samples. Institutions are custodians.

Authorship:

Authorship must be fair.

No ghost authors.

No gift authorship.

E. Research Misconduct:

Misconduct includes:

- Fabrication
- Falsification
- Plagiarism

Institutions must have systems to handle misconduct.

F. Registration:

Clinical trials must be registered in Clinical Trials Registry-India.

G. Collaborative Research:

Agreements must define:

- Data ownership
- Publication rights
- Responsibilities

H. Ethical Review Procedures:

Every research involving humans must be reviewed.

EC reviews:

- Scientific validity
- Risk-benefit ratio
- Consent process
- Compensation plan

Composition:

EC must include:

- Medical experts
- Legal expert
- Social scientist
- Lay person etc as per guidelines

Functions:

- Initial review
- Continuing review
- Monitoring
- SAE review

Registration:

ECs must be registered. Proper record keeping is essential.

I. Informed Consent Process:

Consent is a process, not just a form.

Essential Elements:

- Purpose of research
- Procedures
- Risks
- Benefits
- Voluntary participation
- Right to withdraw

Documentation:

- Written consent preferred
- An impartial witness required for illiterate participants

Waiver of Consent:

Allowed only:

- After EC approval for record-based anonymous data

Re-Consent:

Needed if:

- Protocol changes
- New risks identified
- When a child reaches an age to give consent
- An unconscious patient becomes conscious

Studies involving infertility may need informed consent from both husband and wife.

J. Vulnerability:

Some groups need extra protection.

Vulnerable Groups:

- Children
- Pregnant women
- Economically disadvantaged
- Tribal populations
- Sexual minorities

- Persons with mental illness
- Terminally ill patients

Safeguards:

- Research must address their health needs.
- Extra monitoring required.
- LAR consent when needed.

Children:

Need:

- Parental consent
- Assent from the child

K. Clinical Trials:

Clinical trials test drugs, vaccines and devices.

General Guidelines:

- Follow regulatory rules.
- Ensure scientific validity.
- Register trial.

Special Areas:

- Vaccine trials
- Device trials
- Stem cell trials
- Oncology trials
- HIV trials
- Pregnancy trials

Standard of care should always be one of the arms in a clinical trial. If a placebo is used, then it must be justified. Compensation for injury is compulsory.

Stem cell research may be reviewed by stem cell experts in the IEC.

G. Public health research focuses on communities:

Examples:

- Epidemiological studies
- Surveillance studies

EC must carefully review such cases. Community engagement is very important.

L. Social and Behavioural Sciences Research:

This research studies behaviour and social factors affecting health.

Issues include:

- Stigma
- Cultural sensitivity
- Confidentiality

Qualitative research needs trust and rapport.

M. Human Genetics Research:

Genetic research is sensitive.

Issues:

- Genetic counselling
- Confidentiality

- Family implications
- Misuse of genetic data

Storage of genetic samples needs consent. Gene therapy research needs strict review. Research on embryos requires special safeguards.

N. Biological Materials, Biobanking and Datasets:

Biobanks store samples and data.

Ethical Issues:

- Ownership
- Future use
- Data sharing
- Privacy

Samples must be coded or anonymised. Governance structures must exist.

O. Research During Humanitarian Emergencies:

Disasters create urgent research needs.

Examples:

- Epidemics
- Floods
- Earthquakes

Even in emergencies:

- Ethics must not be ignored.
- Consent must be respected.
- Vulnerable groups need protection.

International collaboration must follow Indian regulations.

ICMR COVID-19 Guidelines:

The COVID-19 pandemic created an unprecedented public health emergency across the world. India also faced serious health, social and economic challenges during this time. There was an urgent need for research. Scientists and doctors had to study the virus, develop treatments, test vaccines and improve public health responses. However, even during an emergency, ethical standards cannot be ignored. To guide research oversight during this crisis, the Indian Council of Medical Research issued special guidance for Ethics Committees reviewing COVID-19-related research.

The purpose of this guidance was to ensure that research during the pandemic remained ethical, scientifically valid and socially responsible. Emergencies create pressure to act quickly. But speed should not reduce ethical safeguards. Human dignity and participant safety must always remain central.

During the pandemic, there was a sudden increase in research proposals. Many studies were related to drugs, vaccines, diagnostics and public health interventions. Ethics Committees had to review these proposals quickly. At the same time, lockdown restrictions made physical meetings difficult. The guidance, therefore, allowed flexibility in review procedures while maintaining ethical standards.

One of the key features of the guidance was the recommendation for expedited review. In urgent public health situations, some research proposals can be reviewed through faster procedures. Virtual meetings, video conferencing and electronic document submission were encouraged. Ethics

Committees could conduct online meetings to avoid delays. However, even expedited reviews must ensure proper risk-benefit assessment and scientific validity.

The guidance emphasised that research must have a strong scientific justification. During a pandemic, weak or poorly designed studies waste time and resources. They may also expose participants to unnecessary risk. Therefore, only scientifically sound research should be approved. The urgency of the situation should not allow low-quality studies.

Informed consent remained a central ethical requirement. However, practical challenges arose during COVID-19. Many patients were isolated in hospitals. Direct contact was limited. Therefore, alternative consent procedures were allowed in specific situations. Electronic consent, telephonic consent or consent through legally authorised representatives were considered acceptable, provided proper documentation was maintained. The aim was to balance infection control with respect for participant autonomy.

Privacy and confidentiality were particularly important during COVID-19. Patients infected with the virus often faced stigma and discrimination. Disclosure of identity could lead to social harm. Researchers had to ensure that personal data was protected carefully. Data sharing for public health purposes had to follow ethical norms and privacy safeguards.

The guidance also addressed the issue of vulnerable populations. COVID-19 disproportionately affected elderly individuals, people with comorbidities and economically weaker groups. These populations required additional protection. Researchers had to ensure that participation was voluntary and not influenced by fear or desperation. Fair selection of participants was necessary to avoid exploitation.

Safety monitoring was another important concern. Clinical trials testing new drugs or vaccines required close monitoring for adverse events. However, lockdowns and healthcare overload made regular monitoring difficult. The guidance allowed flexible monitoring mechanisms such as remote data review and telemedicine follow-ups. Still, participant safety could not be compromised.

COVID-19 research involved collection of blood samples, respiratory samples and other biological materials. Proper biosafety measures were required. Storage and future use of samples had to follow ethical guidelines.

Many institutions were working simultaneously on COVID-19 research. Duplication of efforts should be avoided. Ethics Committees were encouraged to share information and coordinate where possible. Transparency in reporting results was necessary to inform public health decisions quickly.

The pandemic also saw increased use of digital health technologies. Telemedicine consultations and mobile health applications became widespread. Research involving digital data required attention to cybersecurity and privacy protection. Participants should know how their digital data would be used and stored.

If a vaccine or treatment were developed through research, the communities that participated should ideally benefit. Post-research access planning was encouraged. Emergency authorisation concepts were applied during the COVID pandemic.

ICMR - Ethical Guidelines for AI in Biomedical Research and Healthcare:

Artificial Intelligence is increasingly used in healthcare. AI can support diagnosis, predict disease risk and improve decision-making. However, AI also raises ethical concerns. The Indian Council of Medical Research released specific guidelines for AI in healthcare. These guidelines emphasise transparency, accountability and fairness. AI systems must be validated. Bias must be identified and minimised. Data privacy must be protected. Patients must know when AI is being used. There must be human oversight. AI should assist, not replace, clinical judgement. Developers must ensure explainability where possible. Cybersecurity is important. Data breaches must be prevented. Algorithms must be tested before deployment.

Artificial Intelligence (AI) is changing how healthcare works. AI systems can help doctors diagnose diseases, analyse data, predict outcomes, and support clinical decisions. AI can make health services faster and more accurate. It can help in screening, treatment planning and public health monitoring. However, AI also brings new ethical issues, especially when it involves human participants and their data. To guide ethical use of AI, the Indian Council of Medical Research created the first **Ethical Guidelines for Application of Artificial Intelligence in Biomedical Research and Healthcare** in 2023.

These guidelines are meant for everyone who is involved in AI research and applications in health. This includes AI developers, researchers, scientists, clinicians, ethics committees, institutions, sponsors, and policymakers. The purpose is to ensure that AI technology is safe, fair, transparent and respects human rights.

AI systems use data collected from people. This makes data privacy a critical concern. Personal health data is deeply sensitive and must be protected. Researchers must ensure that data is stored securely and used only for agreed purposes. Unauthorised access or misuse of data can cause harm or discrimination. As AI becomes more common in healthcare, systems must be designed to protect privacy at every stage.

An important principle in the guidelines is **accountability**. AI cannot be held responsible for decisions. People must be accountable when AI systems are developed and used. Developers should be transparent about how AI tools work. Clinicians and researchers who apply AI must understand its limitations and take responsibility for its outcomes. Clear accountability prevents harm when errors occur.

AI should also be **trustworthy and fair**. Bias in data and algorithms can lead to unfair outcomes. For example, if an AI model is trained on data from a particular group, it may not predict accurately for other groups. This can worsen health inequalities. Developers and researchers must take steps to detect and reduce bias. They should test AI systems on diverse datasets and assess the fairness of their predictions. Ensuring fairness is essential to protect vulnerable populations and deliver equitable healthcare.

Transparency is another major concern. AI systems, especially those using deep learning, can be difficult to understand. When doctors or patients cannot interpret how AI arrived at a decision, trust is eroded. Explainability should be built into AI tools where possible. Users and patients should understand the basis of decisions, especially when they affect clinical care. Explainability helps clinicians make informed choices and helps patients feel respected.

There is need for **scientific validity and evidence** before deploying AI in real healthcare. AI tools must be rigorously tested for accuracy and safety, just like new drugs or devices. Poorly tested systems can misguide doctors or researchers and cause harm. Ethical review boards and regulators should assess scientific evidence before approving AI systems for research or clinical use.

Autonomy is an important ethical principle. Patients should be informed when AI tools are used in their care. They should know what data will be used and how the AI system may influence decisions. Consent must be obtained when AI uses personal information for research. Consent procedures should be clear and understandable. Patients should have the option to refuse the use of AI in their care if they choose.

AI can pose **safety risks**. Errors in AI predictions can lead to wrong diagnoses or inappropriate treatment. Researchers and developers must build robust systems that minimise risk. Continuous monitoring and testing are necessary even after deployment. Systems should have safeguards and fallback mechanisms so that humans can intervene if an AI decision is questionable.

AI systems learn from data, and the quality of data affects the quality of outcomes. Poor data leads to poor performance. Data must be accurate, complete and representative. Any missing or incorrect data should be identified and corrected before use. High-quality data improves reliability and trust in AI applications.

AI development in healthcare should involve multidisciplinary teams. Clinicians, data scientists, ethicists and legal experts should work together. This collaboration helps ensure that AI tools are technically sound and ethically acceptable. Teamwork also improves understanding of risks and appropriate safeguards.

AI tools should benefit all segments of society and not only well-resourced populations. AI systems should be developed with consideration of socioeconomic and regional differences.

Ethical governance is essential for deploying AI in healthcare. Institutions must develop policies that define how AI will be evaluated, approved and monitored. Governance frameworks should address issues like data sharing, accountability, bias, privacy, and safety. AI hallucinations, biased data, and AI model collapse due to the use of newly generated AI data mean that human original data needs special consideration.

ICH E6(R3) Good Clinical Practice (GCP):

Clinical trials study new medicines. They must protect people's rights, safety and well-being. The ICH E6(R3) guideline updates international standards for how trials should be done. It combines ethics, scientific quality and good clinical practice. It applies from planning to reporting of a clinical trial. This guideline is accepted by regulatory authorities across many countries.

The International Council for Harmonisation (ICH) has developed the Good Clinical Practice (GCP) guideline to establish global standards in clinical trials. The latest version, known as **ICH E6(R3)**, was finalised in 2025 after extensive review and consultation. This guideline represents the most current thinking about how clinical trials should be designed, reviewed and conducted in an ethical and scientifically robust manner.

The core purpose of the ICH E6(R3) guideline is to protect the rights, safety and well-being of people who volunteer in clinical trials. These volunteers deserve respect and care at every step of the research process. Their rights come first, even before scientific objectives and regulatory expediency. The guideline also aims to ensure that clinical trials produce data that are credible, reliable and of high quality. Both ethical considerations and scientific standards are essential. If a study is not scientifically sound, it cannot yield useful results, and participants are subjected to risk without meaningful benefit. Therefore, ethical and scientific standards work hand in hand.

One of the major concepts brought forward in ICH E6(R3) is **risk-based quality management**. Traditional clinical trials involved exhaustive monitoring of all data and procedures. Over time, it became clear that this approach is inefficient and may not improve quality in the most meaningful ways. Risk-based quality management focuses attention on the most critical aspects of a study – those that affect participant safety and data integrity. For example, processes that directly impact safety and outcomes receive focused oversight. This approach allows resources to be used wisely while still ensuring that no important risk is missed.

Another important theme in the guideline is the concept of **quality by design**. Clinical research should not be reactive, responding to problems after they occur. Quality should be built into every stage of a trial from the start. This means that trials must begin with a strong scientific justification, a clear protocol and thoughtful planning. By anticipating risks early in the design phase, researchers can minimise errors and reduce the need for corrective actions later. Quality by design encourages proactive thinking, which strengthens both ethics and efficiency.

Ethics Committees, also known as Institutional Review Boards (IRBs), play a central role in protecting participants. No clinical trial can begin without prior review and approval by an independent committee. The Ethics Committee evaluates the study's scientific rationale, risk-benefit balance, informed consent documents and procedures for protecting privacy. The committee is expected to be multidisciplinary and independent from the research sponsor. Members should include experts in clinical science, ethics, law and community representation. Their work does not end with initial approval; they also monitor ongoing studies and review serious safety events as they arise.

Researchers who conduct clinical trials have clear responsibilities under ICH E6(R3). The person in charge at each site- the principal investigator, must be qualified by training, education and experience to conduct the study. They must follow the protocol closely, ensure that informed consent is properly obtained, and oversee participant safety. Informed consent is more than a form; it is a process of communication in which participants are given understandable information about the study's purpose, procedures, risks, benefits, and their rights. Participants must voluntarily agree to take part without pressure or coercion.

Sponsors are organisations or individuals that initiate, manage and finance clinical trials. Sponsors must ensure that trials are well planned, adequately resourced, and compliant with regulations. They select qualified investigators, provide appropriate training, and implement systems for quality assurance and oversight. Sponsors are also responsible for safety monitoring across all sites participating in a trial. If a potential safety issue arises, the sponsor must act quickly to assess the risk and take protective steps.

Data integrity is a fundamental element of ICH E6(R3). Reliable clinical trial results depend on accurate, complete and consistent data. Data systems must be secure and validated.

Electronic data capture systems, mobile devices and digital tools must function correctly and protect confidentiality. Audit trails should document any changes to data records, who made the changes and why. Protecting participant data from loss, tampering or unauthorised access is essential. Poor data governance may damage trust and render study results unusable.

Closely related to data integrity is the concept of **documentation**. Every step of a clinical trial must be documented. This includes study plans, approvals, consent forms, adverse event reports and final study reports. Clear documentation promotes transparency, accountability and replicability. It also helps investigators and sponsors demonstrate compliance during inspections by regulatory authorities.

The safety of participants is always a primary concern. ICH E6(R3) outlines processes for monitoring adverse events and responding promptly. Serious safety events should be reported quickly to investigators, sponsors and ethics committees. Mechanisms must be in place to provide medical care to participants who experience harm as a result of research procedures.

Non-compliance with protocol or GCP standards poses risks to both participants and data quality. When non-compliance is detected, corrective and preventive actions must be taken. Investigators and sponsors share responsibility for identifying and addressing problems. Over time, patterns of non-compliance can indicate systemic problems that require training, process changes or stronger oversight.

The guideline recognises that modern trials often involve collaborative research sponsored by more than one entity, conducted in multiple countries. Agreements between collaborators should define roles, responsibilities and data ownership. Clear contracts help prevent disputes and ensure that ethical and scientific standards remain consistent across all sites.

ICH E6(R3) also addresses the increasing use of technology in clinical trials, including remote monitoring, digital consent, telemedicine and electronic health records. While technology can improve efficiency, it also raises new ethical and data protection issues. Systems must be tested and secure. Digital consent forms must be understandable and respect privacy. Remote procedures should not compromise ethical safeguards.

The guideline emphasises that ethical review and regulatory compliance are ongoing processes. Changes to study design, procedures or risk profiles require documentation and ethics approval before implementation. Re-consent may be needed if new information emerges that could affect a participant's decision to remain in the study. Many countries follow ICH guidelines and have started the adoption process of the newer E6 R3 version.

New Drugs and Clinical Trials Rules, 2019 & SUGAM Portal:

The Central Drugs Standard Control Organisation (CDSCO) is the regulatory authority responsible for ensuring the quality, safety and efficacy of drugs, vaccines, medical devices and related products in India. Traditionally, regulatory submissions were done in physical form, requiring extensive paperwork, long queues and multiple visits to regulatory offices. CDSCO developed the **SUGAM portal** — a web-based platform where applicants can submit applications, track their status, make payments, and receive approvals electronically.

Clinical trials in India are conducted under the Indian Good Clinical Practice guidelines, the ICMR guidelines, and the New Drugs and Clinical Trials Rules, 2019, in addition to complying with international regulations. SUGAM is an e-governance portal operated by the Central Drugs Standard Control Organisation (CDSCO) to deliver regulatory services for drugs, cosmetics, medical devices, and clinical research. It allows applicants to apply for permissions and approvals online and track their application status.

Hence, it is required that any individual involved in research be well-versed in the latest regulations, both international and national.

References and future reading material:

1. ICMR Guidelines: https://ethics.ncdirindia.org/asset/pdf/ICMR_National_Ethical_Guidelines.pdf
2. ICMR Guidelines for research involving children: https://ethics.ncdirindia.org//asset/pdf/National_Ethical_Guidelines_for_BioMedical_
3. ICMR guideline for Stem Cell Research: https://dbtindia.gov.in/sites/default/files/National_Guidelines_StemCellResearch-2017.pdf
4. Declaration of Helsinki: www.wma.net/e/policy/b3.htm
5. ICH- CGP: www.ich.org
6. FDA GCP:http://www.fda.gov/RegulatoryInformation/Guidances/ucm122049.htm

7. Indian CGP:www.cdsco.nic.in/html/GCP.htm
8. ScheduleY:www.cdsco.nic.in/html/Schedule-Y%20 (Amended%20Version-2005)
9. %20original.htm
10. Clinical Trial Registration: www.ctri.in
11. Central Drugs Standard Control Organisation http://www.cdsco.nic.in/
12. NABH QCI Guidelines for accreditation
13. NewDrugs_CTRules_2019 https://cdsco.gov.in/opencms/export/sites/CDSCO_WEB/Pdf-documents/
14. NewDrugs_CTRules_2019.pdf
15. ICMR COVID guidelines https://www.icmr.gov.in/pdf/covid/techdoc/EC_Guidance_COVID19_06052020.pdf
16. ICMR AI guidelines https://www.icmr.gov.in/icmrobject/custom_data/pdf/Ethical-guidelines/Ethical_Guidelines_AI_Healthcare_2023.pdf
17. ICH GCP E6 R3 version: https://database.ich.org/sites/default/files/ICH_E6%28R3%29_Step4_FinalGuideline_2025_0106.pdf
18. SUGAM is e-Governance system https://cdsco.gov.in/opencms/export/sites/CDSCO_WEB/Pdf-documents/SUGAM_user_manual.pdf

Chapter 2

Scientific Conduct and Research Misconduct

Prof. T. Mohanapriya,
Professor of Surgery, Sri Ramachandra Institute of Higher Education and Research,
Email ID: mohanapriyadr@sriramachandra.edu.in,

Abstract:

Scientific research forms the foundation for advancements in medicine. The integrity of scientific knowledge depends on the strict adherence to ethical principles and responsible research practices. Scientific conduct refers to the standards of integrity, honesty, transparency, and accountability that govern how research is planned, executed, and shared. In contrast, research misconduct is a serious breach of these ethical standards. It undermines the reliability of scientific evidence, public trust in medicine, and patient safety.

This chapter provides an overview of scientific conduct and research misconduct, focusing on the ethical principles behind responsible research practices. It discusses the values of research integrity, outlines good research practices, and highlights the importance of systematic and ethical conduct throughout the research process.

The chapter also covers the types of research misconduct - FFP framework: fabrication, falsification, and plagiarism and about questionable research practices like authorship misconduct, selective reporting, data mismanagement, and "salami slicing." It explores the psychosocial, institutional, and systemic factors that might lead researchers to engage in misconduct, including publication pressure, inadequate mentoring, and insufficient institutional oversight.

The chapter describes the consequences of research misconduct for patients, researchers, institutions, and society. It explains the mechanisms for detecting, reporting, and investigating misconduct, the role of peer review and plagiarism detection tools. It also highlights the importance of institutional ethics committees, regulatory frameworks, and scholarly journals in protecting research integrity.

Finally, it describes the strategies for the prevention of research misconduct, such as ethics education, responsible mentorship, a transparent research culture, and following national and international ethical guidelines.

Keywords:

Ethics, Scientific conduct, Research misconduct, integrity

Objectives:

At the end of this chapter, the medical student should be able to:

1. Define Research integrity, scientific conduct and research misconduct
2. Understand ethical principles in research

3. Understand how to make clear distinctions of violation of ethical standards and make reasonable decisions

4. Differentiate research misconduct from unintentional and honest ethical errors

5. Recognise the specific type of research misconduct

6. Discuss the psychosocial and institutional factors that lead to the occurrence of research misconduct.

7. Understand the consequences of research misconduct on the individuals, patients, research institutions, and society.

8. Learn about detection, reporting, and investigation procedures to be followed in case of research misconduct.

9. Understand the importance of ethics committees, scholarly journals, and regulatory bodies in supporting research integrity.

10. Use research integrity principles appropriately in his or her research and academic work.

Introduction:

Research is the backbone of all the advances in the medical field. Every diagnostic test, drug, surgical procedure, and public health policy is based solely on evidence generated through scientific research. Medical students and Research scholars are the future research guides, and educators must understand how to conduct research and do so ethically. Research misconduct undermines scientific integrity, erodes public trust in medicine, wastes resources and can also harm patients.

In this chapter, we will provide a comprehensive understanding of research misconduct. We have covered the definitions, historical perspectives, types of misconduct, causes and consequences, detection and prevention, and the ethical responsibilities of individuals and institutions. This has been prepared to give practical orientation, emphasise real-world relevance and ethical reasoning and not just regulatory compliance.

Historical Background of Research Misconduct:

Research has always been witnessed as an ethical identity, trust, integrity and honesty of the researcher. But in contraindication, there have been many fraudulent practices in research, which have questioned this assumption in the present research field.

A few such instances in the past are Sir Cyril Burt, a British psychologist accused of fabricating data on intelligence and heredity, the fabrication of cardiovascular research data by John Darsee in the 1980s and the fraudulent autism–MMR vaccine link published by Andrew Wakefield. All of these events faced serious consequences. Events like these question the research integrity and cause harm to society. These incidents not only damaged scientific credibility but also caused direct harm to public health.

In India, the Indian Council of Medical Research (ICMR) and respective institutional ethics committees play a pivotal role in promoting ethical research practices.

Introduction to Research Integrity:

Research is based on honesty and trust. Scientists are expected to present their work without making things up or giving untrue information. They should also give credit to others for their work. Sometimes researchers are under extreme pressure to get funding, incentives and recognition, which can lead to unethical practices.

Scientific conduct is about following standards to maintain public trust in science and research. On the other hand, research misconduct occurs when a researcher intentionally fails to follow these ethical standards. This can include making up data, changing results or taking credit for someone's work and other unacceptable, unethical practices.

Core Values Underlying Research Integrity:

To conduct research in accordance with ethical norms, researchers and institutions must adhere to a few core values. These values include:

- Ethics: treating participants with respect and dignity, respecting their privacy
- Rigour: doing high-quality research
- Relevance: doing research that's meaningful and useful to society
- Transparency: being honest and open about research methods and results
- Respect: respecting colleagues, participants and society
- Impartiality: being objective and unbiased

- Independence: not being influenced by external forces that are not directly involved in the conduct of research like sponsors, funding agencies
- Accountability: taking complete responsibility for all our research work-related issues.

Framework for Good Academic Research Practices:

Research practices follow a certain framework. This framework includes three stages: planning, conducting research and sharing results.

Research Design and Planning:

When planning research, scientists should ensure they have the expertise, facilities, and funding necessary to carry out the project. They should also obtain all necessary approvals and conduct a thorough review of the literature.

- Feasibility: Can the project be done?
- Documentation: Is the plan well-documented?
- Regulatory Approvals: Have all necessary regulatory and ethical approvals been obtained?
- Literature Review: Has the scientist reviewed the existing research on the topic?

Conducting Research:

When conducting research, scientists should document everything carefully and make sure their data is of high quality.

- Data Management: Are data handled properly and are available for others for reference?

- Checklist for Data Collection: Is data collection well-documented?
- Secure Storage: Are data stored safely and securely?

Research Dissemination:

When sharing research results, scientists should choose a medium, such as a peer-reviewed journal. They should also avoid journals that prioritise self-interest over scholarship.

- Choosing a Medium: where will the research be published?
- Avoiding Predatory Journals: Are the journals' metrics and practices reputable?
- Red Flags: Are there any unacceptable issues about the journal?
- Authorship and Credit: Are authors listed in order of their contribution?

Scientific Conduct:

The scientific inquiry is an inseparable part of society's development and health promotion. The rigour, accuracy, and integrity of the research work determine the progress of knowledge. Therefore, research needs to maintain its credibility, and to do so, investigators need to adhere to high standards of honesty, transparency, and strict compliance with ethical guidelines. Various cases of research malpractice have been reported over the last few decades, and there is a need to instil strong ethical principles among research scholars.

The Importance of Scientific Conduct:

Scientific conduct is essential for several reasons. It maintains the integrity of the scientific endeavour, builds public confidence in scientific research, and ensures that society can make empirical decisions based on its results. In addition, strict behavioural codes protect the research participants against harm and deceit.

Fundamental Postulates of Responsible Conduct of Research:

Honesty and Truthfulness:

Researchers must present information and results fully in all circumstances. They should avoid falsification and fabrication of results. Open reporting requires open-minded disclosure of restrictions and null results.

Objectivity and Non-bias:

The investigators must work to reduce bias in study design, data analysis, and interpretation. Bias can stem from vested interests or personal affiliations and thus affect objectivity.

Integrity and Consistency:

Integrity requires one to observe the set protocols and professional guidelines. When these standards are applied consistently, they lead to reliable results.

Transparency and Reproducibility:

Scholarly validation requires transparency. The documentation of approaches and methods of analysis enables one to verify independently and expand on existing knowledge.

Accountability and Stewardship:

Researchers have a responsibility towards funders, participants and the scientific community at large. They have to utilise resources prudently and be stewards of the environment and society.

Respect for Persons, Animals, and the Environment:

Ethical research ensures the safety and well-being of study participants, prioritises their autonomy, minimises harm to animals, and maintains ecological integrity.

Ethical Research - Theories and Frameworks:

Deontological Ethics:

Deontological approaches are focused on duty and rule adherence. In research, strict adherence to consent, protocol approvals, and regulatory laws is mandatory.

Consequentialism:

Consequentialist theories are oriented toward the consequences of actions. Ethical research must seek to maximise benefits and minimise discomfort for public health.

Virtue Ethics:

Virtue ethics predicts character traits such as honesty, diligence, and responsibility. These promote ethical behaviour in any research activity.

Multidisciplinary research:

Different ethical dimensions are important for different disciplines – Biomedical Research emphasises the safety of participants; Social science focuses on Confidentiality and informed consent; Humanities emphasises ethical interpretation and intellectual honesty

Ethical Guidelines:

The International Ethical Guidelines:

International guidelines such as the Nuremberg Code, COPE guidelines, and the Declaration of Helsinki provide comprehensive coverage of ethical principles for conducting research on human subjects.

Indian Ethical and regulatory frameworks:

In India, guidelines on health research are promulgated by the Indian Council of Medical Research. These rules involve participant consent, ethical review procedures, and data protection. University Grants Commission emphasises academic integrity, focuses on plagiarism avoidance and penalises if detected. Funding agencies like DBT, DST and SERB mandate disclosure of conflict of interest, sharing of data and institutional responsibility in maintaining research integrity

RESEARCH MISCONDUCT:

Research misconduct is defined as the breach of a standard or ethical principle in conducting research studies and the violation of a standard or an ethical principle in research studies.

Research misconduct refers to actions by researchers that violate accepted ethical practices and professional requirements.

It is mostly categorised into three FFP frameworks:

Fabrication: modifying the data or findings that are not completely true and claiming that they are real findings.

Falsification: falsifying research materials, instruments or data on purpose to make misleading results, altering the available data, or using inappropriate analysis approaches in order to bias the results.

Plagiarism: copying the work of other people in text, figures or conceptual frames in a piece of work, the act of taking the ideas, techniques, results or language of some other person without giving them the necessary acknowledgement or credit.

It is imperative to distinguish misconduct from unintentional mistakes or intellectual differences; the latter are considered a usual part of the research process and can be corrected.

In short, Fabrication can involve the creation of fabricated laboratory records or fabricated experiment results. Falsification may include cherry-picking or manipulating visuals to make effects appear larger. Plagiarism may include direct copying of text or blurring of ideas without adequate referencing.

Questionable Research Conducts or practices:

Some of the practices might not be against the ethical regulations, but they are ethically questionable includes:

Authorship Misconduct:

Authorship in research work comes as a credit for responsible contribution. According to the guidelines, individuals may be eligible for authorship only if they have played a significant role in the conception, design, execution, or interpretation of the study and are responsible for the content of the manuscript. Violations of standards such as gift or ghost authorship also constitute violations of professional conduct.

Gift authorship: This is assigning authorship to persons who made no substantial contribution to the work.

Ghost authorship: the names of people who have made critical contributions are not mentioned.

Data Mismanagement and Data Misconduct:

Research integrity can only be maintained through proper data management. Poor record-keeping predisposes misconduct. The researchers are expected to have their records of all study activities. Failure to document or share full findings can lead to false information for clinicians and policymakers.

Salami slicing: The practice of turning the results of one research study into several publications.

Selective reporting: not reporting results that are not in line with the hypothesised results.

Such practices compromise the quality of research and falsify the scientific record.

Misconduct during Clinical Research:

Malpractice in clinical research compromises patient safety. Examples include recruiting participants without their informed consent, breaching approved protocols without the required ethical approval, and hiding adverse events. Such contraventions are against the ethical principles.

Reasons and Predisposing Factors of Research Misconduct:

Misconduct is caused by a variety of factors:

Personal factors: the need to publish, the ambition to be recognised, the desire for rapid promotion, the purpose of funding, and a lack of knowledge or training in research ethics.

Institutional reasons: lack of supervision, inadequate mentoring, no clear policies, no adequate monitoring and the inefficient systems of reporting research misconduct.

Systemic: Existing competitive academic settings pressurising for funds, research publications, recognition and rewards for more quantity in research work rather than recognising good quality of research work.

Research Misconduct - Consequences:

Implications of malpractice include several stakeholders:

Patients: access to unsafe treatment, lack of timely, effective treatments, and loss of faith in the healthcare system.

Researchers: publication retractions, loss of educational qualifications, professional consequences and legal or professional penalties.

Institutions: reputational losses, loss of funds, and liability issues.

Society: lack of trust in scientific and medical organisations.

Strategies for the Detection of Research Misconduct:

Peer review: the process is usually not intended to detect fraud, but when reviewers examine the work, they can detect inconsistencies and raise suspicions.

Whistleblowing: reports provided by colleagues, students, and staff on possible misconduct.

Plagiarism detectors: software programs used to detect textual similarities and probable image manipulation.

Research Misconduct Reporting and Investigation:

Organisations ought to create channels for reporting complaints. They should monitor that - Investigations should be fair, transparent, and timely and should also be treated fairly to all the parties. Ethical standards should be upheld, and compliance with protocol should be monitored by ethics committees.

Journals and Publishers' Role in Establishing Research Integrity: Academic journals enhance integrity by establishing guidelines for authorship and disclosure, issuing corrections, retractions, or statements of concern, reporting conflicts of interest, and promoting good publishing practices.

Prevention of Research Misconduct:

Proper training and education in Research ethics is mandatory for students and faculty doing research. Best mentorship promotes professional virtues and integrity in decision-making. Organisations should nurture a culture of integrity rather than productivity.

Research Integrity in India:

In India, the ICMR and the National Medical Commission are some organisations that emphasise the importance of appropriate ethical research practices. Medical colleges will be required to establish ethics committees and provide proper, regular training in research techniques and research ethics. Indian medical students and researchers should understand the ethical guidelines and adhere to them in their research.

Role of Medical Students:

Medical students are obliged to make sure that data collection and reporting is authentic. They are supposed to consult where they are not sure and are bound to report questionable practices using the appropriate institutional channels. Their professional identity will be shaped by the early introduction of rigorous research practices.

Points to Remember:

Scientific conduct is not about following rules, it's about being honest and having integrity. Institutions and researchers must work together to maintain trust in research. Researchers should consult model documents, such as the ICMR National Ethical Guidelines for Biomedical and Health Research, the World Medical Association Declaration of Helsinki and/or the Committee on Publication Ethics (COPE) Guidelines, for further guidance.

Important Checklists for Researchers:

- Planning: ensure study viability. Seek approvals before starting the research study
- Conflict of Interest: disclose financial and professional interests, if any
- Journal Selection: verify the journals' genuineness and peer review process before submitting the research work

By following these guidelines and checklists, researchers can maintain the integrity of research. Scientific conduct and research integrity are crucial to maintaining trust in research and ensuring it is conducted authentically and ethically. Researchers must always prioritise both conduct and research integrity in their work.

References:

1. ICMR National Ethical Guidelines for Biomedical and Health Research.
2. World Medical Association Declaration of Helsinki.
3. Committee on Publication Ethics (COPE) Guidelines.

Exam Questions:

1. Define research misconduct and distinguish it from honest error.
2. Describe the major types of research misconduct with examples.

3. Discuss the ethical principles violated by research misconduct.
4. Explain the role of institutions in preventing misconduct.
5. How can medical students promote research integrity?

Chapter3

Publication Ethics in Research: Plagiarism, Predatory Journals and Predatory Conferences

---

Dr Swati Kumari
Assistant Professor
Department of Microbiology
Sri Ramchandra Medical College & Research Institute
drswatikumari@sriramachandra.edu.in

Abstract:

Publication ethics form the ethical foundation of scholarly communication and are vital for responsible research conduct. In biomedical and health sciences, where published evidence directly impacts clinical decisions and public health policies, ethical publishing is crucial for maintaining scientific credibility and public trust. This chapter offers a comprehensive, exam-focused overview of publication ethics, with targeted discussions of plagiarism, unethical authorship practices, predatory journals and predatory conferences, peer-review ethics, conflicts of interest, and post-publication responsibilities.

The chapter situates publication ethics within the framework of Good Clinical Practice (GCP) and international and national guidelines, emphasising accountability, transparency, and integrity throughout the research process. It examines various forms of plagiarism, including self-plagiarism, image plagiarism, and data plagiarism, as well as detection methods and institutional consequences. The increasing threat of predatory publishing is critically analysed, highlighting its effects on research quality, academic reputation, and evidence-based medicine.

To improve conceptual clarity and exam readiness, real-world case discussions are included to illustrate common ethical dilemmas that PhD scholars and researchers face. This chapter aims to equip doctoral students and early-career researchers with the ethical awareness and practical skills needed for responsible publication and sustained academic integrity.

Objectives:

- To explain publication ethics and their application in biomedical and general research, including Good Clinical Practice.
- To identify and discuss publication misconduct such as plagiarism, unethical authorship, redundant publication, and data manipulation.
- To raise awareness of predatory journals and conferences and distinguish legitimate platforms from unethical practices.
- To apply ethical principles to real research scenarios through case discussions, promoting responsible decision-making in publications.

Section A:

Publication Ethics in Biomedical Research: Principles, Misconduct, and Good Clinical Practice:

A.1. Introduction:

Publication is the final and most visible step in the research lifecycle. In biomedical and health research, ethical publication is not merely an academic requirement but a professional obligation that ensures the integrity of the scientific record, protects public trust, and ensures the responsible translation of research into clinical practice. The increasing emphasis on research output for academic promotion, funding, and recognition has intensified pressures on researchers, sometimes leading to ethical lapses in publication practices. Publication ethics refers to the application of moral principles and professional standards governing the conduct of authors, reviewers, editors, and publishers throughout the process of scholarly communication. Within the framework of Good Clinical Practice (GCP), ethical publication ensures that research involving human participants is reported accurately, transparently, and responsibly, in alignment with national and international ethical guidelines.

A.2. Ethical Foundations of Scientific Publication:

The ethical conduct of publication is grounded in core principles that mirror those of biomedical ethics:

- **Honesty and integrity** in reporting data and findings.
- **Transparency** in methodology, authorship, and conflicts of interest.

- **Accountability** for the accuracy and reliability of published work.
- **Respect for intellectual property** and original contributions.
- **Fairness** in authorship, peer review, and editorial decisions.

International organisations such as the International Committee of Medical Journal Editors (ICMJE), the Committee on Publication Ethics (COPE), and the World Association of Medical Editors (WAME) offer structured guidance to maintain these principles. In India, the Indian Council of Medical Research (ICMR) highlights ethical publication as a natural extension of ethical research practice.

A.3. Authorship Ethics and Contributorship:

Authorship involves both recognition and responsibility. The ICMJE specifies four criteria for authorship: substantial contribution, drafting or critical revision, final approval, and accountability for the work's integrity. Practices such as gift or ghost authorship are deemed unethical if these standards are not met. Contributorship frameworks such as the CRediT taxonomy enhance transparency by precisely documenting each contributor's role.

In the Indian PhD environment, authorship conflicts frequently arise from hierarchical pressures. To avoid such problems, early documentation of contributions, adherence to disciplinary norms, and institutional policies are essential. Examinations often evaluate understanding of how authorship misconduct damages accountability and research integrity.

A.4. Unethical authorship practices:

Gift (Honorary) Authorship: Including individuals without meaningful contribution, often due to hierarchy or influence.

Ghost Authorship: Excluding contributors who substantially participated in the work.

Guest Authorship: To enhance manuscript credibility, such practices distort accountability and violate ethical norms. Ethical authorship requires early discussion, transparency, and documentation of individual contributions.

A.5. Plagiarism and Research Misconduct:

Definition and Types of Plagiarism:

Plagiarism involves using someone else's ideas, text, data, images, or intellectual property without proper acknowledgement. It can take various forms:

- **Direct plagiarism:** copying word-for-word
- **Mosaic or patchwork plagiarism:** Combining copied phrases with original writing
- **Self-plagiarism:** Reusing one's own published work without disclosure
- **Image plagiarism:** Using or altering figures without proper attribution

Plagiarism extends beyond text to include tables, figures, ideas, and data interpretation. The major forms of publication misconduct, along with their ethical implications and institutional responses, are outlined in Table 1.

Table 1. Common Types of Publication Misconduct and Their Ethical Implications

Type of misconduct	Typical manifestations	Ethical implications	Institutional or journal responses
Plagiarism (including self-plagiarism)	Copying text, patchwriting, unattributed paraphrase, undisclosed reuse of one's own work	Misrepresents originality and authorship	Similarity screening, investigation, sanctions
Fabrication	Invented data or results	Undermines truth-seeking	Retraction, institutional inquiry
Falsification	Manipulated images or selective reporting	Distorts evidence base	Correction or retraction
Duplicate submission	Simultaneous submission to multiple journals	Wastes editorial resources	Desk rejection
Redundant publication	Substantial overlap with prior work	Double-counting of evidence	Retraction or notice
Salami slicing	Fragmentation of one dataset	Inflated productivity	Editorial scrutiny

Type of misconduct	Typical manifestations	Ethical implications	Institutional or journal responses
Authorship misconduct	Gift or ghost authorship	Misallocation of credit and responsibility	Institutional mediation
Undisclosed conflicts	Hidden financial or non-financial interests	Bias and erosion of trust	Disclosure or correction
Peer review manipulation	Fake reviewer identities	Subversion of quality control	Retraction
Predatory publishing	Deceptive peer review and metrics	Contamination of literature	Institutional advisories

A.6. Detection and Consequences:

Most journals use plagiarism detection tools like iThenticate as a first screening step. However, similarity reports need contextual interpretation, since acceptable overlap can happen in references, standard terminology, or methodological descriptions. Confirmed publication misconduct may lead to manuscript rejection, retraction of published articles, institutional inquiry, and professional or academic sanctions, depending on severity and intent.

Detection tools and institutional policies:

Similarity detection is a mechanism within a broader integrity regime. The UGC regulations explicitly require higher educational institutions to use technology-based mechanisms, ensure access to plagiarism detection tools, obtain student undertakings of originality, and require supervisor certification; they also specify that institutions must submit soft copies of theses/dissertations to a national repository within a month and create institutional repositories.

The INFLIBNET Centre repository guidance document clarifies that a national electronic theses and dissertations repository, called Shodhganga, is hosted and maintained by INFLIBNET, and that its objectives include improving access, establishing ETD laboratories, and extending access to anti-plagiarism software packages for member universities.

Similarity tools: what they measure and what they do not: Similarity tools compare submitted text to corpora (web, published papers, and institutional databases) and generate a similarity index. Importantly, similarity tools do not determine intent or ethicality. A widely cited discussion of Turnitin stresses that it identifies matched material and produces a similarity index, which is not identical to a conclusion of plagiarism; interpretation must be contextual.

This matters in Indian thesis submissions: universities may treat similarity reports as part of compliance, but the ethical and procedural decision-making must account for exclusions, legitimate quotation, and disciplinary conventions (especially in methods).

The UGC regulations explicitly state that similarity checks should exclude (i) quoted work reproduced with permissions/attribution, (ii) references/bibliography/table of contents/preface/acknowledgements, and (iii) generic terms, laws, standard symbols, and standard equations; it also notes exclusion of common knowledge and coincidental terms up to a limited consecutive-word threshold.

A.7. Peer Review Ethics:

Peer review is the foundation of scholarly publishing and maintaining quality. Ethical peer review involves:

- Confidentiality of submitted manuscripts
- Objectivity and impartiality
- Disclosure of conflicts of interest
- Constructive and timely feedback

Reviewers must not use unpublished information for personal advantage or allow personal bias to influence evaluation. Editors are responsible for ensuring a fair and transparent review process and addressing ethical concerns raised during review.

Post-publication responsibilities include issuing corrections, expressions of concern, or retractions when warranted. The Committee on Publication Ethics emphasises that retractions serve to correct the literature rather than punish authors. Ethical scholarship requires cooperation with these corrective mechanisms.

A.8. Editorial Responsibility and Publisher Ethics:

Editors act as custodians of the scientific record. Their ethical responsibilities include:

- Making unbiased decisions based on scientific merit
- Managing conflicts of interest
- Responding to allegations of misconduct
- Issuing corrections, expressions of concern, or retractions when required

Publishers must support ethical policies, ensure transparency in peer review, and prevent commercial interests from influencing editorial decisions.

A.9. Conflict of Interest and Transparency:

A conflict of interest arises when financial, professional, or personal relationships may influence the conduct or interpretation of research. Ethical publication mandates full disclosure of:

- Funding sources
- Institutional affiliations
- Financial or non-financial interests

Non-disclosure undermines reader trust and may invalidate scientific conclusions.

A.10. Redundant Publication and Salami Slicing:

Redundant publication involves publishing the same or substantially overlapping data without disclosure. Salami slicing refers to dividing a single dataset into multiple minimally publishable units. Both practices misrepresent scientific productivity, waste resources, and distort evidence synthesis. Ethical reporting requires transparency, justification of secondary analyses, and cross-referencing related publications.

A.11. Predatory Journals and Predatory Conferences:

The rapid expansion of open-access publishing has led to the rise of predatory journals and conferences. These organisations focus on profit rather than scholarship and frequently lack authentic peer reviews.

Important Warning Signs to Watch For:

- Guaranteed or rapid acceptance
- Fake impact factors
- Poor editorial transparency
- Aggressive solicitation emails

Publishing in predatory platforms damages academic credibility and undermines scientific integrity.

A.12. Post-Publication Ethics: Corrections and Retractions:

Ethical responsibility extends beyond publication. Errors found after publication should be corrected by:

- **Erratum:** Minor errors
- **Corrigendum:** Author-initiated correction
- **Retraction:** Invalid or unethical research

Retractions are corrective, not punitive, and aim to preserve the integrity of the scientific record.

A.13. Publication Ethics in Good Clinical Practice (GCP):

GCP. represents an international ethical and scientific quality standard for clinical research. The ICH-GCP E6(R3) guideline emphasises participant protection and data credibility, both of which directly affect the ethical permissibility of publication. Similarly, the World Health Organisation's handbook on good clinical research practice integrates ethics, science, and quality assurance. In the Indian regulatory context, ethically compromised study conduct renders subsequent publication ethically untenable, regardless of novelty or impact.

GCP extends beyond the conduct of research to its reporting. Ethical publication under GCP requires:

- Accurate and complete reporting of results
- Respect for participant confidentiality
- Transparency in adverse event reporting
- Avoidance of selective outcome reporting

Failure to publish or to selectively report results constitutes ethical misconduct.

A.14. Case Vignettes for Discussion:

Case 1: Duplicate Submission:

A PhD scholar submits the same manuscript to two journals simultaneously. One accepts the paper, while the other identifies it as a duplicate submission.

Discussion: This violates publication ethics and editorial trust. Manuscripts must be submitted to only one journal at a time.

Case 2: Self-Plagiarism:

An author reuses large portions of methods and discussion from a previous publication without citation.

Discussion: Self-plagiarism is unethical. Prior work must be cited, and text should be rewritten to reflect new contributions.

Case 3: Predatory Conference:

A researcher receives an invitation promising a guaranteed oral presentation and quick acceptance upon payment.

Discussion: This reflects a predatory conference and provides no academic value.

Case 4: Gift Authorship:

A senior faculty member demands authorship despite no involvement.

Discussion: This violates ICMJE authorship criteria and undermines accountability.

A.15. Conclusion:

Publication ethics is an integral component of ethical biomedical research and Good Clinical Practice. Ethical lapses such as plagiarism, authorship misconduct, data manipulation, and predatory publishing erode public trust and compromise scientific progress. Researchers, reviewers, editors, and institutions share collective responsibility for maintaining integrity in scholarly communication.

Education, awareness, and adherence to established ethical guidelines are essential to cultivate a culture of responsible research and publication. Ethical publication is not merely about avoiding misconduct but about upholding the credibility, reliability, and societal value of scientific research.

Section B:

Plagiarism in Academic and Biomedical Writing: Ethical Aspects, Types, Detection Methods, and Prevention Strategies:

B.1. Introduction:

Plagiarism represents one of the most pervasive and consequential ethical challenges in academic and biomedical writing. In an era marked by rapid digital access to information, increasing research output expectations, and intense academic competition, the boundaries between acceptable scholarly use of existing knowledge and unethical appropriation have become increasingly blurred. In biomedical research, where published literature informs clinical decision-making, public health policy, and patient care, plagiarism undermines not only academic integrity but also public trust in science.

Within the framework of GCP, plagiarism is not merely a technical error in citation but a fundamental breach of honesty, accountability, and professional responsibility. Ethical scientific communication requires transparency regarding the origin of ideas, words, data, and images, and demands that originality be clearly distinguished from borrowed intellectual contributions.

B.2. Concept and Meaning of Plagiarism:

Plagiarism is generally understood as presenting someone else's intellectual work—whether ideas, language, structure, data, or creative expression—as your own without proper acknowledgement. It can include copying text verbatim, closely paraphrasing existing material, reusing previously published content, or claiming original ideas without giving credit.

Importantly, plagiarism is an ethical violation independent of legal considerations. While copyright infringement concerns legal ownership, plagiarism concerns the misrepresentation of authorship and the violation of scholarly trust. Even material that is freely accessible or not protected by copyright may still be plagiarised if used without acknowledgement.

Plagiarism can occur across all forms of academic output, including theses, dissertations, journal articles, conference presentations, grant proposals, and teaching materials.

B.3. Historical Perspective and Changing Views on Originality:

Historically, imitation and replication played an accepted role in learning and scholarship, particularly in pre-modern academic traditions where memorisation and reproduction of authoritative texts were encouraged. Over time, especially with the emergence of concepts such as authorship, originality, and intellectual property, plagiarism came to be regarded as unethical and unacceptable.

Modern academic culture places a premium on originality, creativity, and individual intellectual contribution. Within this context, plagiarism is viewed as a form of academic dishonesty that distorts scholarly merit and undermines the credibility of the scientific enterprise.

B.4. Types of Plagiarism:

Plagiarism is not a single uniform act but encompasses several distinct forms, varying in intent and severity.

4.1 Plagiarism of Ideas:

This occurs when an individual uses another person's original concept, hypothesis, or interpretation without acknowledgement. In research, plagiarism of ideas is particularly serious because it deprives the original thinker of intellectual credit and falsely inflates the plagiarist's contribution.

4.2 Direct or Verbatim Plagiarism:

Direct plagiarism involves copying text word-for-word from a source without quotation marks or citation. This form is easily identifiable and often detected through similarity-checking software.

4.3 Mosaic or Patchwork Plagiarism:

In mosaic plagiarism, text is constructed by combining phrases, sentences, or structures from multiple sources with minor modifications. Although the text may appear rewritten, its intellectual framework remains copied.

4.4 Self-Plagiarism:

Self-plagiarism refers to the reuse of one's own previously published material without disclosure. This includes duplicate, redundant, and excessive text recycling. While limited reuse of standardised descriptions (e.g., methods) may be unavoidable, transparency and citation are essential.

4.5 Image and Data Plagiarism:

Using figures, tables, images, or datasets from other sources without permission or attribution constitutes plagiarism. Manipulation of images or selective reuse of data may also cross into scientific misconduct.

4.6 Intentional and Unintentional Plagiarism:

Plagiarism may be intentional, such as deliberate copying, purchasing manuscripts, or submitting ghost-written work. It may also be unintentional, resulting from poor paraphrasing, inadequate understanding of citation practices, or language difficulties.

Regardless of intent, plagiarism remains ethically unacceptable. Authors are responsible for ensuring that their work meets ethical standards of originality and attribution.

B.5. Causes and Contributing Factors:

Several factors contribute to plagiarism in academic and biomedical research:

- Pressure to publish for promotion and career advancement
- "Publish or perish" academic culture
- Easy access to online literature
- Inadequate training in research writing and ethics
- Time constraints and workload stress
- Language barriers among non-native English speakers

These factors highlight the importance of preventive strategies focused on education and mentorship rather than relying solely on punishment.

B.6. Detection of Plagiarism:

Plagiarism detection tools are widely used by academic institutions and journals to screen submissions. These tools compare submitted text against extensive databases to generate similarity reports.

However, similarity scores require careful interpretation. Not all overlap constitutes plagiarism. Common phrases, references, and standard methodological descriptions may produce acceptable similarity. Final determination depends on informed academic judgment rather than numerical thresholds alone.

Similarity-detection software such as Turnitin and iThenticate is a screening aid, not an arbiter of misconduct. The UGC regulations define exclusion criteria and similarity thresholds, while emphasising due process through departmental and institutional academic-integrity panels. Proactive similarity checks, documentation of revisions, and transparent citation practices are the safest compliance strategies for PhD scholars.

The UGC regulations explicitly state that similarity checks should exclude (i) quoted work reproduced with permissions/attribution, (ii) references/bibliography/table of contents/preface/acknowledgements, and (iii) generic terms, laws, standard symbols, and standard equations; it also notes exclusion of common knowledge and coincidental terms up to a limited consecutive-word threshold.

Procedural workflow for similarity reports (a defensible PhD practice): A thesis- and manuscript-safe workflow (aligned with UGC logic)

Step 1: Pre-check (draft stage). Run similarity before final formatting so plagiarism is treated as writing-quality remediation, not cosmetic "score reduction."

Step 2: Apply exclusions correctly. Ensure quotations are correctly marked with citation; make sure references and headers are formatted appropriately so exclusions operate as intended.

Step 3: Investigate high matches ("top-hit audit"). Open the largest matches and classify them: legitimate quotation, properly cited paraphrase, methods boilerplate, or problematic reuse.

Step 4: Remediate ethically. Rewrite in your own analytic voice, add citations for ideas, and reduce reliance on source structure. For self-plagiarism risk, cite earlier work and explain novelty (cross-reference to "Plagiarism taxonomy").

Step 5: Documentation. Preserve: similarity report versions, change log, authorship contributions, supervisor certification, and undertakings. This is not bureaucracy; it is a defensible record if questioned later.

Step 6: Final check and deposit compliance. Ensure the final thesis meets institutional similarity thresholds and repository submission requirements (e.g., Shodhganga/INFLIBNET procedures).

Key Takeaways (Detection and policies)

The UGC framework is not only a "percentage rule"; it is a due-process governance model (exclusions → levels → DAIP/IAIP inquiry → penalties) combined with infrastructure duties (training, tools, undertakings, repositories).

B.7. Consequences of Plagiarism:

The consequences of plagiarism vary according to severity and institutional policy, but may include:

- Rejection or withdrawal of manuscripts
- Retraction of published articles
- Academic disciplinary action

- Loss of degrees, funding, or employment
- Damage to professional reputation

In biomedical research, plagiarism also threatens institutional credibility and public confidence in scientific evidence.

The regulations quantify plagiarism into levels: Level 0 (up to 10%), Level 1 (>10% to 40%), Level 2 (>40% to 60%), and Level 3 (>60%).

They define structured handling: suspected plagiarism is reported to the Departmental Academic Integrity Panel (DAIP), which investigates and submits recommendations to the Institutional Academic Integrity Panel (IAIP). The DAIP is constituted at the departmental level, and the IAIP operates at the institutional level; both are required to follow principles of natural justice, and time-bound reporting is specified.

Penalties differ for theses/dissertations versus academic and research publications. For thesis/dissertation submission, Level 1 requires revision within a stipulated period not exceeding 6 months; Level 2 involves a 1-year debarment from submitting a revised script; Level 3 may result in cancellation of registration for that program.

For staff publications, sanctions include withdrawal of manuscripts and restrictions on increments and supervision rights, depending on severity and repetition.

The different forms of plagiarism and their associated ethical concerns are summarised in Table 2.

Table 2: Common Forms of Plagiarism and Ethical Implications

Form of Plagiarism	Description	Ethical Concern
Idea plagiarism	Use of concepts without credit	Intellectual dishonesty
Direct plagiarism	Verbatim copying	Misrepresentation
Mosaic plagiarism	Patchwork copying	Deceptive authorship
Self-plagiarism	Reuse of own work	Redundant publication
Image/data plagiarism	Uncredited reuse	Scientific misconduct

B.8. Plagiarism and Good Clinical Practice (GCP):

GCP emphasises integrity, transparency, and accountability throughout the research process, including publication. Plagiarism violates these core principles by misrepresenting authorship and distorting the scientific record. Ethical publication under GCP requires accurate reporting, appropriate attribution, and respect for intellectual contributions.

Failure to uphold these standards may compromise evidence-based medicine and patient safety.

B.9. Prevention of Plagiarism:

Effective prevention of plagiarism requires a proactive and educational approach:

- Training in research ethics and scientific writing
- Emphasis on understanding sources before writing
- Encouragement of original synthesis rather than reproduction
- Proper citation and referencing practices
- Use of plagiarism detection tools before submission
- Transparent disclosure of overlap with previous work

Institutions play a critical role by fostering a culture of integrity, providing mentorship, and establishing clear ethical policies.

B.10. Conclusion:

Plagiarism is a serious ethical violation that undermines the foundations of academic and biomedical scholarship. In an increasingly competitive and digitally connected research environment, maintaining ethical standards requires sustained commitment from authors, institutions, reviewers, and editors. While detection tools aid identification, true prevention lies in education, ethical awareness, and responsible mentorship.

Embedding plagiarism on plagiarism within research methodology and Good Clinical Practice curricula is essential to ensure that future researchers uphold the values of honesty, originality, and accountability that underpin scientific progress.

Section c:

Predatory Journals and Predatory Conferences: An Emerging Threat to Research Integrity:

C.1. Introduction:

The integrity of scientific communication relies on transparent editorial processes, rigorous peer review, and ethical dissemination of research findings. In recent years, however, the academic publishing ecosystem has been increasingly compromised by the rise of predatory journals and conferences. These entities exploit the open-access publishing model and academic pressure to publish, offering rapid publication or presentation opportunities without adhering to accepted scholarly standards. Their proliferation poses a serious threat to the credibility of research, evidence-based medicine, and public trust in science.

Predatory publishing is particularly concerning in biomedical and clinical research, where flawed or unvetted findings may influence patient care, policy decisions, and future research directions. Understanding the characteristics, causes, and consequences of predatory journals is therefore essential within the framework of publication ethics and GCP.

Predatory publishing refers to deceptive practices in which journals or conferences charge fees without providing legitimate editorial or peer review services. The Think. Check. Submit. initiative provides a widely accepted framework for identifying such entities. Red flags include unverifiable peer review claims, misleading metrics, aggressive solicitation, and lack of transparency.

C.2. Definition and Concept of Predatory Journals:

Predatory journals are publications that charge authors fees while failing to provide the essential editorial and publishing services associated with legitimate scholarly journals. These services include transparent peer review, qualified editorial oversight, ethical publishing practices, long-term archiving, and reliable indexing.

Predatory conferences are closely related entities that operate on similar profit-driven models. They often invite researchers to present papers or serve as speakers without proper abstract review, academic scrutiny, or involvement of recognised scientific bodies.

While open-access publishing itself is a legitimate and valuable model, predatory journals misuse it by prioritising financial gain over scholarly quality.

C.3. The Historical Rise of Predatory Publishing:

The phenomenon of predatory publishing gained prominence in the early 2010s, coinciding with the rapid expansion of open-access publishing and digital dissemination of research. As funding agencies and institutions increasingly encouraged open access to research outputs, opportunistic publishers emerged, offering fast publication with minimal oversight.

The term *predatory journal* was introduced to describe journals that deliberately deceive authors by mimicking legitimate publishing practices while abandoning ethical standards. Over time, these entities expanded rapidly, often adopting journal titles resembling established publications, falsely claiming indexing status, and listing editorial board members without their consent.

Predatory conferences soon followed as an extension of this business model, targeting researchers with promises of international exposure, keynote opportunities, and certificates of participation.

C.4. Common Characteristics of Predatory Journals:

Predatory journals and conferences share several distinguishing features:

- Absence or superficial peer review
- Guaranteed or unusually rapid acceptance
- Aggressive solicitation through unsolicited emails
- Misrepresentation of indexing, impact factor, or editorial board
- High publication or registration fees with unclear justification
- Broad or vague journal scope lacking scientific focus
- Poor website quality, grammatical errors, and unclear contact details

These features are often deliberately designed to mislead inexperienced or pressured researchers.

C.5. Why Researchers Fall Victim to Predatory Publishing:

Several factors contribute to the continued success of predatory journals:

C.5.1 Academic Pressure:

The "publish or perish" culture places immense pressure on students, early-career researchers, and faculty to demonstrate productivity for promotion, funding, or degree completion.

C.5.2 Lack of Awareness:

Many researchers, particularly trainees and scholars from low- and middle-income countries, lack formal training in publication ethics and journal evaluation.

C.5.3 Deceptive Practices:

Predatory publishers use persuasive language, false metrics, and flattering invitations to create an illusion of legitimacy.

C.5.4 Career Incentives:

In some cases, authors knowingly submit to predatory journals to quickly increase publication counts, raising ethical concerns regarding questionable research practices.

C.6. Predatory Conferences: An Extension of the Problem:

Predatory conferences operate using similar deceptive strategies. They often:

- Invite participants as "keynote speakers" without review
- Accept abstracts with minimal or no evaluation

- Use prestigious-sounding titles such as "World" or "Global" conferences
- Organise meetings primarily for profit rather than scientific exchange
- Offer certificates, awards, or publication opportunities for additional fees

These conferences undermine the purpose of academic meetings, which is to foster genuine scholarly discussion and collaboration.

C.7. Consequences of Predatory Publishing:

The impact of predatory journals and conferences extends beyond individual authors:

7.1 Scientific Consequences:

- Dissemination of flawed or unreliable research
- Contamination of the scientific literature
- Difficulty in conducting valid systematic reviews and meta-analyses

7.2 Professional Consequences:

- Damage to the author reputation and credibility
- Loss of institutional trust
- Barriers to future publication in legitimate journals

7.3 Clinical and Public Health Risks:

In health sciences, unvetted findings may influence clinical decisions, potentially leading to misdiagnosis or inappropriate treatment.

C.8. Ethical Implications under Good Clinical Practice (GCP):

Good Clinical Practice emphasises integrity, accountability, and transparency throughout the research lifecycle. Publishing in predatory journals violates these principles by:

- Misrepresenting peer review and editorial scrutiny
- Undermining accurate reporting of research
- Distorting the evidence base used in healthcare decision-making

Intentional submission to predatory journals may be considered a **questionable research practice**, even if it does not meet strict definitions of fabrication or falsification.

C.9. Identifying and Avoiding Predatory Journals:

Researchers can protect themselves by adopting careful journal-selection practices:

- Verifying indexing claims through trusted databases
- Evaluating editorial board authenticity
- Reviewing peer-review policies and timelines
- Consulting mentors or institutional guidelines
- Using structured checklists, such as journal-assessment tools
- Avoiding unsolicited invitations promising rapid publication

Institutions should actively educate researchers and integrate publication ethics into research training programs.

C.10. Institutional and Global Responses:

Academic institutions, funding bodies, and professional organisations play a critical role in combating predatory publishing. Strategies include:

- Strengthening research ethics education
- Establishing clear publication policies
- Encouraging quality over quantity in academic evaluation
- Promoting awareness of legitimate indexing platforms
- Supporting transparent open-access publishing models

Legal actions against deceptive publishers have demonstrated that predatory practices can be challenged, though enforcement remains complex given their global, often opaque operations.

C.11. Conclusion:

Predatory journals and conferences represent a significant and evolving threat to the credibility of scientific research. By exploiting academic pressures and gaps in awareness, these entities undermine peer review, distort scientific communication, and compromise evidence-based practice. Addressing this challenge requires a multifaceted approach involving education, ethical leadership, institutional accountability, and responsible publishing practices.

Within the framework of publication ethics and Good Clinical Practice, researchers must recognise that ethical responsibility extends beyond conducting research to ensuring its appropriate and trustworthy dissemination. Upholding these principles is essential to safeguarding the integrity of science and maintaining public confidence in research.

References:

1. University Grants Commission. Promotion of Academic Integrity and Prevention of Plagiarism in Higher Educational Institutions Regulations, 2018. New Delhi: UGC.
2. Indian Council of Medical Research. National Ethical Guidelines for Biomedical and Health Research Involving Human Participants. New Delhi: ICMR; 2017.
3. International Committee of Medical Journal Editors. Recommendations for the Conduct, Reporting, Editing, and Publication of Scholarly Work in Medical Journals. Updated 2024.
4. World Health Organisation. Handbook for Good Clinical Research Practice. Geneva: WHO; 2005.
5. International Council for Harmonisation. Guideline for Good Clinical Practice E6(R3). 2025.
6. Committee on Publication Ethics. Retraction Guidelines. COPE; 2019.
7. Office of Research Integrity. Avoiding Plagiarism, Self-Plagiarism, and Other Questionable Writing Practices. ORI; 2015.

Chapter 4

Open Access Publishing and Ethics in Digital Research

Dr. Divyambika CV
Professor, Department of Oral Medicine and Radiology
Sri Ramachandra Dental College and Hospital
SRIHER (DU), Chennai -600116
Email: cvdivyambika@sriramachandra.edu.in

Abstract:

The chapter titled *Open Access Publishing and Ethics in Digital Research* explores the transformative impact of digital technologies on scholarly communication and the evolving ethical challenges within this landscape. Digital research, encompassing tools such as artificial intelligence, machine learning, electronic health records, and online data repositories, has significantly enhanced data accessibility, research efficiency, and global dissemination of knowledge. Concurrently, open access (OA) publishing has emerged as a pivotal model to democratize scientific information by enabling unrestricted access to research outputs, thereby promoting equity, collaboration, and increased citation impact.

However, this rapid digital expansion raises critical ethical concerns, including issues of data privacy, informed consent in virtual environments, secondary data use, and cybersecurity risks. The chapter highlights the importance of adhering to fundamental ethical principles—autonomy, beneficence, non-maleficence, and justice—while integrating emerging concepts such as explicability in artificial intelligence. It also critically examines the rise of predatory publishing, emphasising the need for vigilance and adherence to standards set by organisations such as COPE and DOAJ to maintain research integrity.

Further, the role of Institutional Ethics Committees (IECs) is underscored in ensuring ethical compliance, particularly in digital and data-intensive research contexts. Frameworks such as FAIR data principles and DECIDE model are presented as essential tools for responsible data sharing and ethical decision-making. The chapter concludes by advocating for harmonised global regulations, transparent research practices, and proactive ethical governance to balance innovation with accountability. Overall, it provides a comprehensive overview of how ethical rigour must evolve alongside technological advancements to sustain trust and credibility in modern scientific research.

Keywords:

Open access publishing, Digital research ethics, Data privacy, Predatory journals, FAIR data principles

Introduction:

Digital publishing includes the propagation of information through multiple channels, such as infographics, blogs, eBooks, video, online abstracts, audio, and through different channels, such as websites, email services, podcasts, mobile applications, and social media. The advent of laptops, tablets and smartphones has provided ready, instant access to information released through these digital platforms. [1] The origin of digital publications can be dated back to 1971, when the first digital version of the American War of Independence was created. Soon after, a digital version of 60,000 books was published. The emergence of CD-ROM technology, the introduction of e-books in diverse formats and PDF-based e-books further enhanced the digital research ecosystem. The rise of electronic health records (EHR) and the internet in the late twentieth century paved the way for advanced digital health innovations such as telehealth services and online patient portals. The advent of smartphone technology further enhanced accessibility to e-books and the advanced formats such as HTML, XML, ePub, and cross-platform applications, further aiding the broader dissemination of scholarly information. These digital platforms have accelerated the speed of publication and widened the global visibility, thereby disseminating the research findings to a larger network of diverse populations. However, there are quite a few challenges associated with digital platforms in terms of the publication of non-validated, non-peer-reviewed preprints online for immediate visibility, thereby compromising the research standards and ethics. The shift in the trend towards faster and immediate availability of such preliminary observations and outcomes has occurred during the COVID era, when urgent treatment and clinical decisions had to be made in a short time. Thus, alterations in research design, guarded peer-review processes, methodological modifications and standardisation undermined the research standards and ethical norms, thereby challenging the informational value and clinical relevance. (2)

Open access publishing refers to free and instant availability of scholarly evidence to the researchers and clinicians across the globe. This sharing of data among the scientific communities, helps them not only in updating the latest developments, but also preventing the unnecessary duplication of work. The subscription-based model, on the other hand, allows access for the institutions/resources settings who are able to cover the subscription costs. (3) The current chapter highlights the ethical dimensions of open access publishing and funding; ethical issues associated with digital research. highlighting key considerations for maintaining integrity and fairness in the scholarly communication landscape.

Overview of digital research:

Digital research involves the use of the digital technological advancements in diverse capacities. The digital methodological tools include the use of Artificial Intelligence (AI), machine learning (ML), 3D design, digital ethnography, online surveys, hardware and software applications to develop and implement novel research methodologies. Large-scale data is efficiently processed and managed using secure cloud-based, remote storage tools. These digital technologies may function as objects of study, such as the investigations into blogs, social networking platforms, virtual worlds, online communities, and instant messaging environments. In addition, the digital environment can constitute the context or setting of research, providing access to data sources such as online datasets and repositories, search engines, data aggregation platforms, and automated data-scraping mechanisms. The major benefits offered by the digital research is faster analysis, better data accessibility, thereby offering better avenues to study the human behaviours and different components of biomedical research. The common digital research services include analysis of humanities data, social media, network analysis, geospatial research and better visualisation complex large-scale data.[4] Thus, digital research facilitates creation of new knowledge across diverse disciplines through data collection, analysis, visualisation and publication.

Advanced technologies in the digital healthcare system, namely electronic health records, telemedicine (teleoncology, teleradiology, telepathology, telepharmacology), wearable health devices (Eg: fitness trackers, smartwatches, and insulin pumps), artificial intelligence applications, and the emergence of smart hospitals have been significantly striving to produce better patient outcomes in a more cost-effective manner. Integration of digital health over the recent years has enhanced accessibility and efficiency with more personalised care. However, these technological advancements have inherent challenges, including data privacy concerns, cybersecurity vulnerabilities, and disparities in access to digital technologies, thereby posing barriers to implementation and adoption across different communities. The key concerns include data privacy and security, disparities in access, and the definitive need for evidence-based validation of digital interventions. Thus, the fundamental challenge revolves around integration of digital health technologies within real-world clinical environments, such that these digital health solutions are feasible, secure and offer benefits to the patients and healthcare providers. [5]

Open Access Publishing: Concepts and Models:

Open access (OA) publishing allows scholarly research to be freely and immediately accessible online without restrictions to readers worldwide, bypassing subscription paywalls to maximise visibility and impact. The key models are Gold, Green, Hybrids, Diamond, and Bronze access journals. These models help enable widespread research publication and reuse. Online access to OA publications is free and comes with copyright and licensing details. The principle of open access is that the author pays for the publication as article processing charges (APCs), which removes the financial barriers for the readers to access the publication. Public access to articles increases their visibility, usage, and impact on citations. Gold open-access publications make the article freely available on the publisher's website and are supported by APCs. Green open access is also known as self-archiving, in which authors deposit a version of their manuscript before publishing (preprint) for a specific time. Hybrid open access enables authors to pay an APC to make their individual articles open access, while the others can be accessible only to subscribers. Diamond or platinum open access models do not charge APCs to authors or the readers. It is the most inclusive and equitable type of open access. Bronze open access models allow the readers to access the publications after an embargo period. Also, the content will be restricted to subscribers or pay-per-view.

Benefits of Open Access Publishing:

Open access encourages fair access to knowledge, which is especially advantageous for researchers, students, independent scholars, and institutions in low- and middle-income countries. OA makes it easier for people to adapt and implement research in their local contexts and promotes more equitable global knowledge sharing when combined with multilingual abstracts, plain-language summaries, and easy-to-read formats. Research from a variety of fields has shown that open access articles have more downloads and frequently receive more citations than their paywalled counterparts, particularly in fields that are fast-paced and applied. In addition to scholars, this unfettered access enables the public, educators, practitioners, politicians, NGOs, and media to interact with scientific findings. Openly accessible research promotes interdisciplinary utilization and international collaboration, minimizes redundancy in efforts, and fosters the creation of innovative ideas and achievements. The exposure of academic institutions, research centers, and funding organizations that embrace open access is increased by OA publishing. The OA enables a wider use of the study findings in industry, healthcare, policymaking, and classrooms. The San Francisco Declaration on Research Assessment and other initiatives encourage evaluating scholarship based on its inherent merit rather than publication prominence. Additional strategies to realign incentives toward rigour and practical utility include the disclosure of unfavourable outcomes, portable review reports, and open peer review.

Ethical foundation of open access publishing:

Publications and journals play a pivotal role in academic career. The move in favor of open access publishing is a significant advent in the academic publishing world. Conventional journals based on subscription are afflicted from it raises questions about the economics of sharing knowledge. By making research free of cost, open access publishing can fasten scientific breakthroughs and decrease redundant efforts.[(6)] In the context of enhancing transparency, accountability and reproducibility, globally acclaimed bodies such as the United Nations Educational cultural and scientific Organisation (UNESCO) can engage key stakeholders, which includes the institutions, funding agencies, research communities, peer-reviewed journals, and the wider public, to develop and promote international standards for transparent, reproducible, and meaningful research practices. These efforts can build upon existing frameworks that define research transparency and provide practical tools, such as the FAIR Guiding Principles (Findability, Accessibility, Interoperability, and Reusability), which guide effective scientific data management and stewardship. [7]

Authorship and contributorship are among the most pivotal, sensitive, and intricate areas of academics and thus demand critical thinking among the authors, editors, and readers. The International Committee of Medical Journal Editors (ICMJE) has established four criteria for authorship. These include: (1) Considerable contribution (making substantial contributions to the conception/ design/acquisition/analysis/ interpretation of data of the study); (2) Critically Revising of work (critically evaluating and modifying the manuscript for enhancing the scientific and intellectual content); (3) delivering final approval (providing final approval of the manuscript version which would be published); and (4) accountability (agreement of being accountable for all aspects of the work, ensuring that issues related to the accuracy or integrity of any part of the study are adequately examined and addressed.)[8]

Authors have an ethical responsibility to conduct and report research with honesty and integrity. This includes being transparent and morally responsible in all aspects of the research process, such as hypothesis testing, laboratory procedures, and the collection, analysis, and interpretation of data. Authors must ensure that their findings are reported accurately and without any manipulation or falsification of data. Researchers must remain vigilant about potential conflicts of interest that may influence the conduct or reporting of research. They should avoid entering into agreements with individuals, companies, government agencies, or funding bodies that could pressure them to modify or adjust research outcomes to align with specific agendas or expectations. Journal editors often receive numerous manuscripts for consideration to be published each year, and the decision to publish often relies primarily on the evaluations provided by peer reviewers. Reviewers have a responsibility to provide objective, constructive, and confidential feedback directly to the editor rather than addressing comments to the authors. Additionally, reviewers should submit their evaluations within the stipulated timeframe, typically within three to four weeks after receiving the manuscript. If they are unable to meet this deadline, they must inform the editor in advance so that appropriate alternate arrangements can be made for the peer review process. (9)

Predatory publishing and ethical pitfalls:

Predatory journals tremendously afflict research fields such as food, health, and well-being, and impact the population big time. Predatory scientific journals are those that are dubious, equivocal, parasitic, illegitimate, perfidious, counterfeit, garbage, deceitful, and dark. Predatory journals frequently attract submissions by sending aggressive, unsolicited invitations to researchers, often encouraging them to publish work, including work outside their specific area of expertise. Organisations such as the Committee on Publication Ethics (COPE), the Directory of Open Access Journals (DOAJ), and the Open Access Scholarly Publishing Association (OASPA) play an important role in promoting ethical publishing practices and maintaining quality standards in scholarly communication and research publications. COPE is a membership organisation dedicated to educating and supporting editors, publishers, universities, research institutions, and others involved in publication ethics. DOAJ is a community-curated online directory that indexes and provides access to high-quality, peer-reviewed open-access journals. OASPA represents a global community of organisations engaged in open scholarship and promotes open access as a primary model for the dissemination of scholarly outputs.

To ensure credibility and transparency, journals must maintain high standards in their content and operations. The published material should be original, clearly presented, and free from ambiguity and plagiarism. Journal websites should be regularly updated and properly maintained, with adequate security measures in place to protect users from potential threats such as viruses or malware. Journals are also expected to adhere consistently to their declared publication schedule and frequency unless exceptional circumstances arise. Furthermore, journals should clearly outline their policies for electronic backup and long-term digital preservation of published content, particularly when the journal or publisher ceases operations. If certain content is not freely accessible, the terms of access, such as registration, subscription, or pay-per-view fees, should be transparently stated on the journal website. Similarly, if offline versions (such as print editions) are available, this should be clearly described along with any associated costs. In addition, journals should maintain a qualified editorial board or advisory panel composed of recognised experts in the journal's subject areas. The journal's website should also provide complete information about its editorial leadership, including the full names and institutional affiliations of editors, as well as contact details for the editorial office, including a valid mailing address.

Ethics in Digital Research:

Digital ethics guidelines are rapidly evolving. Around 160 guidelines have been curated in the past 5 years for many fields. [10] Among them, medical ethics remains the most well-established in both research and clinical settings. [11] Most of the work follows an ethical framework known as principlism, which provides general principles to guide ethical decision-making. [12]Core ethical principles: autonomy, beneficence, non-maleficence, and justice. Tom Beauchamp & James Childress have proposed four principles of ethics: Beneficence, Non-Maleficence, Autonomy, and Justice. These are used and taught within clinical practice and research ethics, and sometimes the fifth principle of Explicability is also integrated. [13] The first principle, autonomy, emphasises recognising every individual as possessing inherent moral value and respecting their capacity to make independent decisions. It requires that the choices or actions of an autonomous individual should not be limited without valid and justifiable reasons. However, the concept of ethical relativism, which denies the existence of a single universal moral standard, can make it challenging to justify the application of fixed moral principles. Non-maleficence, the second principle, concerns the obligation to avoid causing harm to oneself or others and to prevent pain, suffering, or offence. When viewed through an ethical relativist lens, researchers must exercise particular caution in interpreting what constitutes harm within the specific sociocultural context in which the ethnography is conducted. Beneficence refers to reducing, or preventing harm and to promoting benefits to advance the welfare of individuals and communities. It indicates the necessity to understand that the community defines what is good and normal, instead of applying their own standards. Justice, the fourth principle, concerns the fair distribution of benefits and harms and the use of equitable procedures in making distributive decisions. Researchers must critically examine how justice is defined in the community under study, explicitly reflect this understanding in their work, and demonstrate ethically sound practice. The artificial intelligence research community has proposed a fifth principle: explicability. This highlights the intelligibility and accountability, which enable and operationalise the other ethical principles. [(14)]

Informed consent in digital and remote research settings:

eConsent has become increasingly important in health research, particularly during and following the COVID-19 pandemic. Keeping the research sites remote, these systems aid in generating quantitative and qualitative data that are challenging to maintain in paper-based consent. Despite the increasing use of eConsent, ethical review processes remain variable. This becomes tedious when committees must evaluate diverse multimedia formats such as graphics, audio, video, podcasts, and interactive web interfaces. [(15)] The setback with eConsent is that it is harder for participants to fully understand the study and make their own independent decision. This finding underscores the need to build a standardised framework that incorporates guidelines such as the Nuremberg Code, the Declaration of Helsinki, and the Belmont Report. [(16)]

Ethical challenges in secondary data use and data repurposing:

In secondary data use, researchers revisit existing data and examine it from a new angle to answer a question, rather than collecting new data. [17] The main problem with secondary data use is that it might harm participants and necessitate renewed consent. If the data is completely anonymous, it means no one can tell who the participants are. If the researcher cannot identify any participants, the risk to participants is very low. Hence, a full ethics committee review may not be necessary. In such cases, the researcher can request a waiver of consent, meaning they do not need to obtain consent again from the participants. [18] There are lots of controversies in repurposing data that would mainly focus on protecting the rights of individuals whose data is being used. Important rights include privacy and autonomy.[19] Ethical issues with respect to digital technologies are still in the nascent phase, and the implementation of these considerations across geographies is a major challenge.

Data Privacy, Confidentiality and Security:

By sharing research data from health care systems, we can accelerate the progress of data through secondary use. However, sharing of such information intrudes into sensitive public information and carries the risk of re-identification of patients. Hence, frameworks have been formulated to assess the risk of re-identification and mitigate it. Regardless of whether the records are correct, the total number of re-identifications equals the number of records identified. [20] One critical focus in the present scenario of globalisation is the efficient documentation and filing of data. As business complexity increases, it becomes necessary to support overall operational effectiveness. In this context, BPAD ((Badan Perpustakaan Arsip dan Dokumentasi) Malang), is a system which is a system which is expected to document all messages, both incoming and outgoing files. It helps in the collection, management and control of data in the form of a database and data analysis to draw up a program of activities.[21]

The General Data Protection Regulation (GDPR), which came into force on 25 May 2018, establishes distinct roles in data governance, including data controllers, data processors, and data protection officers (DPOs). The data controller is responsible for overseeing and maintaining records of all activities related to data processing and may designate one or more data processors to collect and process data on its behalf. The Data Protection Officer plays a crucial role in ensuring that the organization handles and processes personal data in full compliance with the requirements of the GDPR. The principles included in data protection include, fairness, transparency, lawfulness, limitation of purpose, Minimisation of data, accuracy of data, limited storage, integrity, confidentiality and accountability.

"The Health Insurance Portability and Accountability Act of 1996 (HIPAA)" was enacted by the US Congress to revise the "Internal Revenue Code of 1986". to enhance portability and continuity of health insurance coverage, and to simplify the administrative processes associated with health insurance. The primary aim of the legislation is to reduce the misuse of healthcare insurance and delivery, and extend the medical coverage and enhance access to long-term healthcare services

Ethical Issues in Emerging Digital Technologies:

Digitaltechnologieshavenowbecomeintegratedintotheeveryday lives of individuals and organisations, posing significant ethical concerns for society regarding privacy, data security, fairness, protection from online harms, transparency, and accountability. It is necessary to address the ethical considerations in digital technologies to deliver broader and equitable social benefits. The well-established digital technologies, such as smartphones, robotics and AI, are increasingly governed by certain guidelines or industry self-regulation. In parallel, regulatory frameworks have been introduced or are under development to oversee digital platforms and related domains, including data protection and online safety. Examples include platform-focused legislation within the European Union, comprehensive data privacy regulations such as the GDPR, and national laws addressing online harms, such as Germany's NetzDG in Germany.

Though these digital technologies offer significant advantages in boosting the economy and improving productivity across diverse sectors, they also entail inherent disadvantages and limitations with respect to data privacy. Some of the notable examples of breaches in data privacy include the Cambridge Analytica scandal, in which 50 million Facebook users' personal data was acquired without their consent, and concerns surrounding facial recognition technologies, arising from potential racial bias embedded within algorithms, which may result in discriminatory impacts on specific racial or ethnic groups. (22)

Ethical issues identified in different digital technologies, namely cloud services, robots, IoT, and AI, share overlap with respect to data privacy, and hence may not be unique for individual technologies. Since algorithms and data ware being used in most of these platforms and applications, AI holds the key to the guidelines developed for these technologies. Cloud computing services and Software as a Service (SaaS) models have raised important ethical considerations regarding the shared informational responsibilities between hosting companies and service providers. These responsibilities include safeguarding consumer privacy, ensuring service reliability, regulating data mining practices, and clarifying issues related to data ownership. While extensive government restrictions may not always be necessary, certain sectors such as banks, law firms, and hospitals may require stricter regulatory oversight due to the sensitive nature of the data they handle. The word "blockchain", which was frequently used in finance related to cryptocurrencies, has started appearing in research papers related to ethics. However lacunae still exists regarding ethics of blockchain and understanding its potential role and socio-technical challenges. With respect to devices, the Digital Services Act package, a draft legislative framework proposed by the European Union in December 2020, aims to regulate large digital platforms, often referred to as "structuring platforms." The proposal seeks to introduce measures that promote fair competition and protect users. For instance, it could prohibit practices such as the mandatory pre-installation of certain applications on mobile phones and computers, as well as the automatic imposition of specific application stores, such as those operated by Apple or Google.

Academic institutions have played a key role in advancing discussions on the ethics of developing and using robots, particularly from 2006 to 2008. In 2017, the United Nations Educational, Scientific and Cultural Organisation (UNESCO) published the COMEST Report on Robotics Ethics, which examined the ethical implications of using robots across multiple sectors, including industry, the military, transportation, healthcare and welfare, education, households, agriculture, and environmental management. The report highlighted several ethical challenges and provided recommendations related to robotics governance. These included the need for workforce retraining, the promotion of public dialogue on the societal impacts of robotics, the importance of environmental impact assessments, and the expansion of ethical discussions to include emerging technologies such as the Internet of Things (IoT). Some ethical subjects related to robotics include autonomy, decision-making, learning, the legal status of robots, security, and data protection.

Artificial intelligence: Guidelines and recommendations:

Following the report titled AI for Europe in 2018, the European Commission released the Ethics Guidelines for Trustworthy Artificial Intelligence in April 2019. A group of independent experts developed the guideline framework after getting feedback from more than 500 contributors. The main aim of these guidelines is to encourage the development and application of "Trustworthy Artificial Intelligence," which refers to AI systems that operate in a lawful, ethical, and reliable manner. The guidelines are intended for all stakeholders involved in the design, development, deployment, implementation, and use of artificial intelligence, including companies, organisations, researchers, public services, government agencies, institutions, civil society organisations, workers, consumers, and individuals who may be affected by AI technologies.

In April 2021, the European Commission introduced a proposal outlining new rules and actions to promote "excellence and trust in Artificial Intelligence." This initiative adopts a risk-based regulatory approach for the governance of AI systems. Under this framework, AI applications are categorised according to their level of risk. Systems considered to pose an unacceptable risk are proposed to be banned, while those classified as high risk are subject to strict regulatory obligations. AI systems with limited risk must comply with specific transparency requirements. Most AI applications, however, are expected to fall into a fourth category—minimal risk—and will therefore not be subject to significant regulatory oversight.

However, more recently in 2020, an international initiative was launched by France and Canada known as The Global Partnership on Artificial Intelligence (GPAI), with support from several countries and regions, including India. The partnership brings together experts from diverse stakeholders, including civil society, industry, governments, and academia, to promote the responsible design, development and use of AI. It also facilitates collaboration on AI governance, the ethical use of data, and the funding and advancement of innovative ideas in artificial intelligence. Though numerous guidelines and frameworks have been put forth for AI-related research, Europe and the US are the early adopters of integrating ethics in digital research. However, Mexico, Japan, Singapore, and the UAE have also laid out guidelines to promote ethics in AI-related research.

Institutional Ethics Committees and Digital Research:

Institutional Review Boards and Ethics Committees are independent bodies established to protect the rights, safety and well- being of research participants. Their core value is to ensure the research methodology follows autonomy, beneficence, non-maleficence, justice and confidentiality. The board typically composed of scientific members(Clinicians and researchers), non-scientific member, legal or ethics advisor/representative, human right activist and layman. This diversification helps in the balance of the participant protection. By critically reviewing study protocols, risk–benefit ratios, informed consent processes, and data privacy measures, IRBs/ECs shape research quality and integrity. Their oversight promotes ethically sound study designs, safeguards vulnerable populations, enhances public trust in research, and ultimately strengthens the credibility and societal value of scientific research.[(23)]

The key pointers of an IRB/EC are:

- Ethical Gatekeeping
- Participant Protection
- Ongoing Oversight

The ethical review of digital protocols and open data sharing balances transparency against participant privacy. The boards assess how digital data is collected, stored, analysed and shared to ensure compliance with consent, confidentiality and data-protection regulations by safeguarding against re-identification, misuse and unauthorised access. [(24)] With the rapidly expanding digital-research methodologies, the traditional randomised control trials are too slow and rigid; they need modern solutions like simulation-based studies and real-world evidence to provide timely, robust, cost- effective valuations while ensuring the protocols by adapting to the digital health technologies.[(25)]

Responsible Data Sharing and Reuse:

Authors Alther and Gonzalez et al. have eloquently debated on the growing demand for transparency and reproducibility, implying the importance of data sharing as a core obligation. Yet they also question data ownership and the protection of participant confidentiality, fearing misuse or a lack of credit for data creators. This could be delineated by informed consent, disclosure risk assessments, de-identification, restricted access when necessary, and governing the shared digital data. Key highlights of the article include the importance of documentation and transparency, highlighting the role of metadata, codebooks, version control, and data provenance in making shared data meaningful and reusable. The authors also advocate that research data and analytical code should be recognised as scholarly products, deserving formal citation and academic credit similar to traditional publications. [(26)]

The FAIR Data Principles, introduced in 2016, provide a set of guidelines aimed at improving the "Findability, Accessibility, Interoperability, and Reusability" of data in digital research and other scholarly assets. Under these principles, Findability requires that data be easily discoverable by both humans and computer systems. This is achieved through the use of rich, machine-readable metadata and the deposition of datasets in searchable and well-recognised repositories. Accessibility ensures that once data are located, they can be retrieved by authorised users through standardised communication protocols. Interoperability emphasises that data should be structured to enable integration with other datasets and facilitate analysis using advanced computational tools, such as machine learning and artificial intelligence. Finally, Reusability requires that datasets include clear usage licenses, detailed provenance information, and adherence to community- or discipline-specific data standards to enable future use and reproducibility. [(27)]

Best Practices and Recommendations:

The DECIDE framework gives a structured approach to support ethical decision-making for digital behavioural data. As always, the ethical issues arise after the deed is done, i.e., after publication. Hence, the DECIDE encourages a proactive, continuous ethical reflection across all the stages of a research study rather than a one-time approval. It guides researchers in critically examining consent, privacy, data sensitivity, potential harms, and the misuse of digital data by providing guiding questions, frameworks, flowcharts, etc. It not only guides the researchers but also the IRB/EC by promoting responsible, transparent and ethically sound digital behavioural research. An iron-clad ethical framework that takes into account the rapidly developing digital era, as researched by the IRB/EC, will help guide researchers, peer reviewers, and editors in publishing high-quality, transparent, and ethically sound digital research while minimising unnecessary delays in the review and publication process. [28]

Future Directions:

The ethical norms in open sciences are evolving from static compliance to continuous, reflexive ethical oversight. With the expansion of digital and open data, scholars emphasise proactive ethics that anticipate privacy risks, secondary data misuse and downstream harms. The advantages of making data findable, accessible, interoperable, and reusable are evident, despite the difficulties in implementation and enforcement. The scientific community can improve the transparency, reproducibility, and impact of research by encouraging strict data management procedures and collaboration among researchers, librarians, publishers, and repositories. The ongoing initiatives by institutions such as the NIH, AGU, and Worm Base provide excellent examples of how to incorporate FAIR principles into scientific publishing and research.[29]

Global regulations are being harmonised in practice through a few specific mechanisms that improve consistency in cross-border research and data sharing, rather than becoming "one single law". Regulators in clinical research are increasingly aligned on common standards, such as ICH Good Clinical Practice (GCP). According to the EMA, ICH E6 GCP is an international standard that facilitates the mutual acceptance of clinical trial results across significant regulatory regions and supports a unified framework. The EU uses adequacy decisions to determine whether a non-EU nation offers a "sufficient level" of protection for privacy and data. Adequacy allows personal data to move between jurisdictions without requiring additional security measures, thereby harmonising transfer regulations. International organisations are clearly advocating for the harmonisation of standards, governance, and regulatory strategies in AI and digital health. Harmonised regulatory frameworks and cogent governance are presented in the WHO's Executive Board report as crucial pillars for secure and successful digital transformation in health systems. Global coalitions that develop common technical and policy frameworks are the driving forces behind harmonisation in genomics and health data. The GA4GH Framework specifically seeks harmonised methods based on human rights (privacy, non-discrimination, fairness) to facilitate responsible international sharing of genomic and clinical data. International requirements are being pushed by major funders. Establishing de facto alignment in research practice, the NIH Data Management & Sharing Policy sets guidelines for data management and sharing planning (effective 2023) that institutions implement with consideration for participant privacy and consent.[30]

The incorporation of ethics through frameworks and governance in the digital technologies provided by private companies will benefit consumers and offer diverse benefits to society. Making ethical practices visible to consumers through transparency and accountability not only helps build trust but also encourages suppliers to adhere to ethical standards, ensuring the acceptance and use of their products. Users of digital services and the technologies that support them may also encounter ethical challenges related to self-responsibility and decision-making. Increasing awareness of ethical issues through education and improved data literacy is essential for empowering users to make informed choices. Some of the key challenges include coping with the rapid evolution of technology, different cultural perspectives across countries, states and enterprises acting both as judges and parties to the ethical framework. Industry support for ethics frameworks and self-regulatory initiatives may sometimes be intended to avoid stricter formal regulations. This can also lead to "ethics washing," where companies exaggerate their commitment to ethics and social responsibility to gain public trust and profits, while failing to implement these policies effectively internally.

Conclusion:

Together, digital research and open access publishing signify a revolutionary change in the production, sharing, and use of academic knowledge. Open access models raise ethical issues with quality control, predatory publishing, authorship accountability, and funding disparities even as they improve equity, visibility, and international cooperation. At the same time, strong ethical oversight is required to protect participant autonomy, privacy, data security, and justice due to the quick development of digital research methodologies, from artificial intelligence to secondary data reuse. Maintaining trust and integrity in digital scholarship requires upholding fundamental ethical principles, which are backed by frameworks like FAIR data governance, and proactive ethical review mechanisms. Harmonised international regulations, responsible data stewardship, and improved institutional ethics frameworks will be essential as open science develops to make sure that research transparency benefits society without sacrificing ethical rigour.

References:

1. Bhatia VK. Challenges and future directions in digitally mediated research publication and dissemination. InDigital Scientific Communication: Identity and Visibility in Research Dissemination 2023 Dec 30 (pp. 311-326). Cham: Springer International Publishing.

2. Barroga E, Matanguihan GJ. Fundamental shifts in research, ethics and peer review in the era of the COVID-19 pandemic. Journal of Korean medical science. 2020 Nov 23;35(45).

3. Parker M. The ethics of open access publishing. BMC medical ethics. 2013 Mar 22;14(1):16.

4. Tsatsou P. Digital technologies in the research process: Lessons from the digital research community in the UK. Computers in Human Behavior. 2016 Aug 1;61:597-608.

5. Shapoo N, Shapoo N, Rehman A, Boma N. Smart Healthcare: The Role of Digital Health in Modern Medicine. Health Care Sci. 2025 Jun 1;4(3):179-187.

6. Michael Parker. The ethics of open access publishing; Parker BMC Medical Ethics 2013; 14:16

7. Winker MA, Bloom T, Onie S, Tumwine J. Equity, transparency, and accountability: open science for the 21st century. The Lancet. 2023 Oct 7;402(10409):1206-9.

8. Khattri MB, Subedi M, Pandey R, Bhandari P. Authorship and Contributorship in Publication Ethics and Guidelines: The Publishers' Perspective. Dhaulagiri Journal of Sociology and Anthropology. 2025 Dec 31;19(2):1-6.

9. Carraway LN. Ethics for and responsibilities of authors, reviewers and editors in science. The American Midland Naturalist. 2009 Jan;161(1):146-64.

10. Watch A. AI ethics guidelines global inventory. Algorithm Watch. 2020 Apr;30.

11. Peters D, Vold K, Robinson D, Calvo RA. Responsible AI—two frameworks for ethical design practice. IEEE Transactions on Technology and Society. 2020 Feb 18;1(1):34-47.

12. Nyrup R. From general principles to procedural values: responsible digital health meets public health ethics. Frontiers in Digital Health. 2021 Jul 2; 3:690417.

13. Floridi L, Cowls J. A unified framework of five principles for AI in society. Machine learning and the city: Applications in architecture and urban design. 2022 May 21:535-45.

14. Hair N, Akdevelioglu D, Clark M. The philosophical and methodological guidelines for ethical online ethnography. International Journal of Market Research. 2023 Jan; 65(1):12-28.

15. Yusof MY, Teo CH, Ng CJ. Electronic informed consent criteria for research ethics review: a scoping review. BMC Medical Ethics. 2022 Nov 21;23(1):117.

16. Alifia RR, Sadeghi M, Eluru M, Jafari M, Grando MA. Bridging ethical gaps in digital health research: a framework for informed consent aligned with NIH guidance. BMC Medical Ethics. 2025 Oct 8;26(1):132.

17. Szabo V, Strang VR. Secondary analysis of qualitative data. Advances in nursing science. 1997 Dec 1;20(2):66-74.

18. Tripathy JP. Secondary Data Analysis: Ethical Issues and Challenges. Iran J Public Health. 2013 Dec;42(12):1478-9.

19. Green S, Hillersdal L, Holt J, Hoeyer K, Wadmann S. The practical ethics of repurposing health data: how to acknowledge invisible data work and the need for prioritization. Medicine, Health Care and Philosophy. 2023 Mar;26(1):119-32.

20. Sweeney L, Yoo JS, Perovich L, Boronow KE, Brown P, Brody JG. Re-identification Risks in HIPAA Safe Harbor Data: A study of data from one environmental health study. Technology science. 2017 Aug 28;2017:2017082801.

21. . Putri MA, Trihapningsari D, Hapsani AG, Putri CS. Data Encryption and Security in Data Storage Management Information System Using Blowfish Algorithm. MATICS: Jurnal Ilmu Komputer dan Teknologi Informasi (Journal of Computer Science and Information Technology). 2024 Sep 23;16(2):92-6.

22. Cadwalladr C, Graham-Harrison E. Revealed: 50 million Facebook profiles harvested for Cambridge Analytica in major data breach. The guardian. 2018 Mar 17;17(1):22.

23. Mehta P, Zimba O, Gasparyan AY, Seiil B, Yessirkepov M. Ethics committees: structure, roles, and issues. Journal of Korean medical science. 2023 Jun 26;38(25).

24. Lvovs D, Creason AL, Levine SS, Noble M, Mahurkar A, White O, Fertig EJ. Balancing ethical data sharing and open science for reproducible research in biomedical data science. Cell Reports Medicine. 2025 Apr 15;6(4).

25. Guo C, Ashrafian H, Ghafur S, Fontana G, Gardner C, Prime M. Challenges for the evaluation of digital health solutions—A call for innovative evidence generation approaches. NPJ digital medicine. 2020 Aug 27;3(1):110.

26. Alter G, Gonzalez R. Responsible practices for data sharing. Am Psychol. 2018 Feb-Mar;73(2):146-156.

27. Vita R, Overton JA, Mungall CJ, Sette A, Peters B. FAIR principles and the IEDB: short-term improvements and a long-term vision of OBO-foundry mediated machine-actionable interoperability. Database (Oxford). 2018 Jan 1;2018:bax105.

28. Shaw H, Brown O, Hinds J, Nightingale SJ, Towse J, Ellis DA. The DECIDE Framework: Describing Ethical Choices in Digital-Behavioural-Data Explorations. Advances in Methods and Practices in Psychological Science. 2025;8(3).

29. Alves T. FAIR data: what it is and how we can support its principles. Science Editor. 2024 Jun 23;47(3):110-2.

30. Thaldar D, Uberoi D, Thorogood A, Milne R, Newson AJ, Hall A, Glazer D, Esselaar P, Joly Y. Communicating clearly about data sharing in genomics. Human Genomics. 2025 Jul 14;19(1):80.

Chapter 5

Publication Misconduct

Dr.Linga devi Thanasekaran
Coordinator of Centre for Professional Development
SRIHER
Institutional Ethics Member for both Undergraduates and postgraduates
Email id : drlinga2@gmail.com

Objectives:

At the end of the chapter research scholars will be able to

- Explain the concept of publication misconduct and its types.
- Understand authorship ethics and misconduct and analyse authorship issues appropriately.
- Recognise and manage Conflicts of interest in publishing in accordance with accepted ethical guidelines.
- Understand the responsibilities of authors, editors, and reviewers involved in scholarly publishing.
- Be able to use Plagiarism software and AI responsibly and effectively.
- Interpret the historical milestones that have shaped policies and frameworks related to publication ethics.

Abstract:

Publication ethics forms the foundation of credible work by research scholars. In an increasingly competitive academic environment driven by publication metrics, publication misconduct has emerged as a significant concern globally and within India. This chapter provides a structured overview of publication misconduct, regulatory frameworks such as the Committee on Publication Ethics (COPE) and the International Committee of Medical Journal Editors (ICMJE), and institutional responsibilities in preventing unethical practices. It further examines conflicts of interest, authorship criteria, the use of AI in publishing, post-publication corrections and appeals, and illustrative examples from international and Indian cases. Emphasis is placed on fostering a culture of research integrity through education, transparency, and responsible use of technological tools.

Keywords: Publication ethics, misconduct, plagiarism, authorship, conflict of interest, software tools, research

1. Introduction:

Scientific publication is the primary mechanism through which research findings are communicated to the academic community and the public. Misconduct in publication practices affects the transparency, accountability and reproducibility of scholarly research.

Publication misconduct may take several forms, including plagiarism, falsification or fabrication. Publication misconduct has increased globally, including in India, largely due to insufficient awareness of ethical publishing standards, rising academic pressure, and growing reliance on publication metrics for career advancement. In response to these challenges, several international organisations have developed guidelines to promote ethical publication practices. Prominent among these are:

Committee on Publication Ethics (COPE), International Committee of Medical Journal Editors (ICMJE), World Association of Medical Editors (WAME)

University Grants Commission (UGC), in India, introduced the Promotion of Academic Integrity and Prevention of Plagiarism Regulations (2018)

2. Types of Publication Misconduct (FFP):

The three primary forms of misconduct are collectively known as FFP:

F for Fabrication, F for Falsification, P for Plagiarism

a. **Fabrication**: Fabrication refers to inventing or creating fictitious data or results that were never actually obtained during research. Examples include: Inventing experimental data, creating fictitious survey responses, and reporting results from experiments that were never conducted.

b. **Falsification:** Falsification refers to manipulating data, the methodology and the research process. **Examples include** altering statistical results and modifying images or graphs. Falsification distorts research findings and leads to incorrect scientific conclusions.

c. **Plagiarism:** Plagiarism refers to the use of another person's intellectual work without proper acknowledgement. Forms of plagiarism include: direct copying of text, mosaic plagiarism, paraphrasing without citation and self-plagiarism. Most journals use plagiarism detection tools to help them identify textual similarity before proceeding to peer review.Turnitin, iThenticate, and Urkund are used to detect plagiarism.

- Open-source similarity-checking tools are also being used. However, similarity scores must be interpreted carefully, as not all overlap represents plagiarism. It is the duty of the editorial board to ensure that all published articles do not exceed the journal's minimum plagiarism score, follow the guidelines, and take appropriate actions as suggested by the Committee on Publication Ethics (COPE).

  (Tables 1 and 2)

Minor Copying: using short and common phrases that cannot be rephrased (e.g., in the methodology section) is allowed. **Clear Plagiarism:** Unattributed use of a large part of text, ideas, or data is definitely plagiarism. **Self-Plagiarism (Text Recycling):** Re-using a large part of the author's own previous work without attribution is not allowed.

A low score does not guarantee originality, and a high score does not automatically mean fraud, but it does require a detailed human review.

- Other types of publication misconduct are:
  i. Conflict of Interest in Publication
  ii. Redundant /duplicate publication
  iii. Authorship misconduct
  iv. Unethical citation practices
  v. Salami Slicing

3. Conflict of Interest (COI) in Publication:

Conflict of interest (COI) arises when professional, personal, financial or institutional relationships influence the conduct, interpretation, or reporting of research

.ICJME therefore requires full transparency and disclosure of potential conflicts of interest by authors, editors, and peer reviewers.

Proper COI disclosure allows readers and policymakers to evaluate research findings with a clear understanding of potential influences.

Financial	Monetary relationships that may influence research outcomes	Industry funding, consultancy payments
Personal	Personal relationships that may affect objectivity	Family members involved in the study
Academic	Professional competition or collaboration	Rival research groups competing for recognition
Institutional	Affiliations that may influence interpretation of results	Research funded by the investigator's institution

Conflict of Interest Disclosure Workflow in Journals:

Typical journal procedures for managing COI include the following steps:

Manuscript Submission

↓

Authors complete **COI disclosure form.**

↓

The editorial office reviews all the declarations.

↓

Peer reviewers and editors have to disclose conflicts

↓

COI statements published with the article

4. Redundant or duplicate publication:

Publishing the same information in more than one journal without proper disclosure is called duplicate publication. These can mislead readers and introduce bias, especially in systematic reviews and Meta-Analyses.

Predatory Journals: Predatory journals are publications that charge authors publication fees but fail to provide essential editorial and peer-review services. These journals often prioritise profit over scientific quality and may accept manuscripts without proper review. As a result, they contribute to the dissemination of unreliable or low-quality research.

Common characteristics include:

- Lack of rigorous peer review
- Aggressive email invitations requesting manuscript submissions
- Rapid acceptance and publication within an unrealistically short period

- False claims of indexing in reputable databases
- Unclear editorial policies and contact information
- Editorial boards with unverifiable or fake members

Identifying and Avoiding Predatory Journals:

Researchers should take several precautions before submitting manuscripts to journals.

- Verify whether the journal is indexed in recognised databases.
- Examine the editorial board and confirm the authenticity of its members.
- Review the journal's peer-review process and publication policies.
- Check whether the journal follows ethical publishing standards recommended by organisations such as the COPE and WAME
- Consult institutional guidelines or mentors before submitting manuscripts.

Many universities also recommend referring to the UGC-CARE-approved **journal lists** when selecting publication venues.

5. Authorship misconduct:

ICMJE Authorship Criteria:

Individuals should meet the following 4 criteria to qualify as an author

- They should have made substantial contributions to conception or design of work, or acquisition/ analysis/ or interpretation of data for the work

- Either drafted the research work or should have revised it critically
- provided final approval of the version to be published
    - Should agree to be accountable for the research work

If they do not meet the authorship criteria but have contributed to the article, then they can be acknowledged.

Authorship misconduct refers to unethical practices related to the assignment of authorship in academic publications.

a. Gift Authorship: refers to those people whose names appear in the author's list despite not making any contribution to the research. This may be done to gain favour with senior colleagues, supervisors or influential researchers.

Examples include:

- Adding a department head or senior professor who did not participate in the study
- Including colleagues to strengthen academic relationships

b. Honorary Authorship: Honorary authorship involves including an individual as an author based on their reputation, authority, or institutional position rather than their actual contribution to the study.

For example, a well-known scientist may be added as an author to enhance the manuscript's credibility.

c. Ghost Authorship: Refers to those individuals who are not acknowledged as authors despite making substantial contributions to the manuscript preparation or the scientific research.

- Example: Professional writers or statisticians prepare manuscripts but are not credited
- Industry sponsors contribute to the writing of research papers but remain undisclosed

d. Guest Authorship: Guest authorship refers to the inclusion of prominent individuals as authors primarily to increase the likelihood of manuscript acceptance or enhance the prestige of the publication.

e. Purchased Authorship: Purchased authorship occurs when individuals pay money or offer other benefits to be listed as authors on a manuscript without contributing to the research. E.g., paper mills and unethical publishing services.

f. Authorship Order Manipulation: It involves intentionally altering the sequence of authors in a way that misrepresents their contributions. In many disciplines, the first author and the corresponding author receive significant recognition

Contributor Roles (CRediT Taxonomy) to Prevent Authorship Manipulation:

To improve transparency in publishing and prevent authorship manipulation, many journals now require authors to specify each author's individual contributions. One widely accepted system recommended by COPE and ICJME is the **CRediT system (Contributor Roles Taxonomy)**. **The CRediT** system helps to ensure that due credit is given appropriately and that all contributors are acknowledged for their specific roles in the research and publication process.

Major Contributor Roles in the CRediT Taxonomy include:

i. **Conceptualisation-**Development of the research idea, research goals, and design of the study framework.

ii. **Methodology:** Design of the research methods, experimental procedures or analytical approaches used in the study.

iii. **Data Curation:** Management, organisation, and maintenance of research data.

iv. **Formal Data Analysis**

v. **Investigation:** Conducting experiments, data collection, or fieldwork related to the research study

vi. **Original Draft writing**

vii. **Review and Editing** of manuscript

viii. **Visualisation:** Preparation of figures, graphs, charts, or other visual elements that illustrate research findings.

ix. **Supervision:** Oversight and leadership of the research project

x. **Project Administration.**

xi. **Funding Acquisition** for the research project. Many journals now require authors to submit **detailed contribution statements** during manuscript submission, as it promotes fair attribution of credit.

6. Citation Manipulation:

Citation manipulation refers to unethical practices in which references are added to a manuscript primarily to increase citation counts rather than to support the scientific content of the research.

Types of Citation Manipulation:

- **Excessive Self-Citation:** Excessive self-citation occurs when authors repeatedly over cite their own previously published work without clear scientific justification to increase an author's citation metrics and academic visibility.
- **Coercive Citation:** When editors or reviewers pressure authors to add citations to specific articles, often from the same journal, in return for manuscript acceptance.
- **Citation Stacking:** Refers to agreements between two or more journals to cite each other's articles in order to artificially inflate their citation statistics.
- **Citation Cartels:** Involves network groups of researchers, institutions, or journals that cite each other's publications to increase citation counts.
- **Irrelevant Citation Insertion:** Refers to references included in a manuscript even when they are not directly related to the research topic. These citations may be added with the intention of promoting specific authors, journals, or institutions.
- **Citation Padding:** Refers to the practice of adding an excessive number of references that provide little or no meaningful contribution to the study. The intention may be

to increase citation counts for particular articles or to create the appearance of extensive literature support.

7. Salami slicing:

Segmenting or slicing one major study into multiple publishable papers is called salami slicing.

Ethically, to avoid publication misconduct, the research scholars should practice writing information in their own words, cite the references appropriately, read the source article completely and take what is needed, remember to use tools that are free to use and get permission for copyrighted tools too.

Ethical Oversight Committee:

An ethical oversight committee is a fundamental requirement for research involving human participants or animals. Ethical oversight requires researchers to disclose potential hazards, conflicts of interest, and any risks associated with the research procedures.

The committee will ensure that Institutional ethics committee approval and, where appropriate, informed consent have been obtained by the authors prior to the commencement of the study. For experimental or observational studies, authors should obtain approval from the IEC (Institutional Ethics Committee) or the IRB (Institutional Review Board) before starting the study.

For studies involving humans, we must obtain informed consent from participants before they are enrolled. Details of ethical approval, such as the letter from the approving ethics committee and the approval number, should also be mentioned.

Research involving human subjects must comply with the ethical principles set out in the Declaration of Helsinki, adopted by the World Medical Association (WMA). These guidelines emphasise respect for human dignity, protection of participant rights, risk minimisation, and the requirement for ethical review prior to research initiation.

Use Of Artificial Intelligence In Publications:

The rapid adoption of artificial intelligence tools for manuscript preparation, literature synthesis, and language editing has introduced new ethical considerations in academic publishing. While AI tools can support writing and data analysis, they cannot qualify for authorship because they lack accountability and intellectual responsibility.

Authors using AI tools should clearly disclose the name of the AI system used, Specify how the tool contributed to manuscript preparation, ensure human verification of all generated content, avoid using AI for data fabrication, citation generation without verification, or peer review manipulation. Editorial policies from COPE now emphasize that AI should function **only as an assistive tool and not as a substitute for scholarly responsibility.**

Editorial Response To Suspected Misconduct (Flow Chart 1):

Manuscript Submitted

↓

Plagiarism Screening

↓

Peer Review

↓

Suspicion of Misconduct?

/ \

Yes No

↓ ↓

Editorial Inquiry Publication

↓

Author Explanation

↓

Institution Investigation

↓

Correction / Expression of Concern / Retraction

Editorial Screening And Investigation Process For Suspected Publication Misconduct:

When a manuscript is submitted, editors follow a structured screening and investigation process to detect publication misconduct.

Initial Manuscript Screening:

The editorial process begins when a manuscript is submitted to a journal. At this stage, the editorial office conducts a **preliminary screening** to check for

- Completeness of the submitted manuscript
- Adherence to journal formatting guidelines
- Plagiarism similarity reports using plagiarism detection software
- Ethics committee approval for studies involving human or animal participants
- Conflict-of-interest disclosures by authors

If the manuscript fails to meet basic ethical or technical requirements, it may be **rejected without peer review**.

Plagiarism and Similarity Assessment:

Most journals use plagiarism detection tools to screen manuscripts for textual overlap with previously published literature. Editors will carefully interpret similarity reports because not all similarity represents plagiarism; some overlap may occur due to references, methodology descriptions, or commonly used phrases.

If excessive similarity is detected, the editor will may:

- ask for clarification from authors
- ask for manuscript revision
- reject the manuscript in cases of confirmed plagiarism

Editorial Evaluation:

After the initial screening, the editor evaluates the manuscript for scientific relevance, originality, and ethical compliance. At this stage, the editor will decide whether the manuscript should proceed to peer review. Editors will also check for potential **red flags** such as:

- inconsistent or unrealistic data patterns
- image duplication or manipulation
- suspicious authorship patterns
- possible duplication of publication

Peer Review Process:

If the manuscript passes editorial evaluation, it is sent to independent peer reviewers with relevant expertise. Reviewers assess the manuscript's scientific quality, methodology, originality and ethical compliance.

Peer reviewers may also identify potential ethical issues, including:

- plagiarism or duplicate publication
- unethical research practices
- fabricated or manipulated data

Reviewers will report any concerns directly to the editor.

Identification of Suspected Misconduct:

If editors or reviewers suspect publication misconduct, the journal will then initiate a formal investigation process. Editors typically follow ethical guidelines recommended by COPE.

The editor may:

- **Reject the manuscript** if serious misconduct is confirmed before publication
- **Request for revision or correction** if errors are minor
- **Expression of concern** if the investigation is ongoing
- **Article retraction** if misconduct is confirmed after publication

Institutional Investigation:

If serious misconduct is suspected, the editor may notify the author's institution or research ethics committee for a formal investigation. Institutions are responsible for evaluating the conduct of their researchers and determining appropriate disciplinary actions. The journal may temporarily **pause the review or publication process** until the investigation is completed.

Authors, editors, peer reviewers and publishers should disclose conflicts of interest if any.

Responsibilities of the Publisher's commitment to preventing misconduct:

It is the duty of the publisher to oversee all the stages of publishing and is committed to making sure that all the editorial decisions made are completely independent, unbiased and unaffected by any funding sources.

Post-Publication Appeals And Corrections:

Ethical responsibility continues even after publication, and journals should facilitate the post-publication dialogue and correction through letters to the editor and commentaries. Post publication corrections include

- Erratum: minor correction of important mistake or omission that does not have any significant effect on the overall conclusion of the research work.
- Expression of concern – to highlight that there is an ongoing investigation about the article or inform the readers about its unreliability.
- Retraction notice–Major ethical breach, such as unethical scientific work, redundant publication, plagiarism, peer review manipulation, reuse of data without authorisation, data fabrication, and failure to disclose a major ethical breach that would have unduly influenced the research work.

Consequences Of Publication Misconduct:

Publication misconduct can have serious consequences for individual researchers, academic institutions, journals, and the broader scientific community.

Immediate Consequences: Article Retraction-Journals may retract published articles when serious ethical violations or unreliable data are identified. Retraction helps to correct the scientific record and alert readers to unreliable findings. The other immediate consequences are loss of academic credibility, loss of research funding, disciplinary actions by Institutions, blacklisting of authors and legal Implications.

Long-Term Consequences include damage to professional reputation, loss of career advancement, reduced chance of academic collaboration and potential negative impact on future research and erosion of credibility and trust of the public in research and publication practices.

Preventive Measures To Avoid Publication Misconduct:

- Adherence to Ethical guidelines developed by COPE, ICJME, WAME
- Good Research and Medical Practices: Maintaining ethical conduct throughout the research process
- Transparent Data Management
- Use of Plagiarism Detection Tools before submission
- Disclosure of Conflict of Interest
- Submission of manuscripts in carefully selected reputable journals

Timeline: 1998–2023 Historical Milestones In Publication Misconduct:

The following documented examples are widely cited in publication ethics literature and have contributed to reforms in editorial oversight, institutional governance, and ethical training.

Indian cases:

Anil Potti (2010-2012), a cancer researcher in the United States, was involved in high-profile falsification and misinterpretation related to a genomic predictor of cancer treatment.

Ranjit Kumar Chandra (1990s – 2000s)-a nutrition researcher of Indian origin working abroad, fabricated clinical trial data related to infant nutrition and immune function.

Authorship and plagiarism cases in Indian Universities (2016-2019)- several Indian universities reported cases of plagiarism involving theses and journal publications, which influenced the enforcement of UGC Promotion of Academic Integrity and prevention of plagiarism regulations in 2018.

International Cases:

Andrew Wakefield publication (1998)-Vaccine –Autism controversy- linking data misinterpretation of vaccines to autism, **Hwang Woo-suk (2004–2006)-a Stem cell Researcher** involved in fabrication of experimental data related to human embryonic stem cloning, **Jan Hendrik Schön (2002)** a physicist, found to have fabricated and reused data, **Diederik Stapel (2011)**a social psychologist, admitted to fabricating data in over 50 publications, **Yoshitaka Fujii (2012)** an anaesthetists, who fabricated clinical trial data and **Paolo Macchiarini's (2014–2018)** work on synthetic tracheal transplants was found to involve misrepresentation of clinical outcomes and ethical violations.

2021-2023 Paper Mills and Organised Publication misconduct:

Large-scale investigations revealed that international publishers had identified production services involving fabricated data, manipulated images, and False authorship, leading to the retraction of hundreds of articles. (Table 3)

Conclusion: Publication ethics ensures transparency and credibility in research. Fabrication, falsification, and plagiarism are the most serious forms of publication misconduct. Authors, editors, reviewers, and publishers have a shared responsibility for maintaining publication integrity. We have to remember that technological tools assist in detecting publication misconduct but cannot replace human judgment.

By following these practices, researchers can protect the integrity of their work and contribute to responsible scientific publishing.

References:

1. COPE. Retraction Guidelines (2019).

2. ICMJE. Recommendations for the Conduct and Publication of Research (2023). International Committee of Medical Journal Editors. Defining the Role of Authors and Contributor

3. UGC. Promotion of Academic Integrity and Prevention of Plagiarism Regulations (2018).

4. Retraction Watch Database (Accessed 2016–2023).

5. COPE Council. COPE Discussion document: Artificial intelligence (AI) in decision making — English 2021 Sept 24

6. COPE Council. COPE position - Authorship and AI – English. 2023

7. Publication misconduct: Perceptions of participants of a faculty development programme Suman P Singh1, Shashi K Dhir2, Monika Sharma3, Tejinder Singh4 https://nmji.in/publication-misconduct-perceptions-of-participants-of-a-faculty-development-programme/

Table 1: Comparative Overview – FFP vs Conflict of Interest vs Redundant Publication

Parameter	Fabrication / Falsification / Plagiarism (FFP)	Conflict of Interest (COI)	Redundant / Duplicate Publication
Definition	Core research misconduct involving data invention, manipulation, or unattributed copying	Undisclosed personal, financial, or institutional relationships influencing research	Publishing substantially overlapping data in multiple venues without disclosure
Nature of Violation	Direct distortion of scientific record	Compromised transparency and objectivity	Distortion of evidence base through repetition
Intent	Often deliberate (may occasionally be reckless)	May be intentional (non-disclosure) or negligent	Often strategic to increase publication count
Impact on Evidence Base	Produces false knowledge	Creates interpretive bias	Skews systematic reviews and citation metrics

Parameter	Fabrication / Falsification / Plagiarism (FFP)	Conflict of Interest (COI)	Redundant / Duplicate Publication
Detection Mechanism	Statistical review, image forensics, plagiarism software	Disclosure forms, institutional review	Editorial cross-checking, database similarity screening
Regulatory Guidance	COPE retraction guidelines; ICMJE authorship accountability	ICMJE disclosure standards; COPE flowcharts	COPE redundant publication guidelines
Possible Conse-quences	Retraction, blacklisting, funding loss, institutional action	Correction, disclosure statement, editorial sanction	Retraction, publication ban, institutional warning
Example Cases	Wakefield; Hwang Woo-Suk; Stapel	Undisclosed pharma funding cases	Salami slicing in clinical datasets

Table 2: Fabrication vs Falsification vs Plagiarism (Internal FFP Comparison)

Feature	**Fabrication (F)**	**Falsification (F)**	**Plagiarism (P)**
Definition	Making up data or results	Manipulating data or images	Using other people's ideas or words without attribution
Data collection/ analysis/ manuscript Stage when it occurs	Data collection stage	Data analysis/ reporting stage	Manuscript preparation stage
Ways to detect it	Statistical improbability patterns	Image manipulation software; raw data mismatch	Similarity detection software
Effect on Research Validity	Completely invalidates findings	Distorts conclusions	Misrepresents intellectual ownership
Categori-sation of misconduct	Serious scientific misconduct	Serious scientific misconduct	Academic misconduct (may escalate to research fraud)

Feature	Fabrication (F)	Falsification (F)	Plagiarism (P)
Corrective Action	Retraction + institutional inquiry	Retraction + disciplinary action	Rejection or retraction; mandatory correction

Table 3 Historical Timeline

Year	Event	Nature of Misconduct	Regulatory Impact
1998	Andrew Wakefield vaccine-autism paper	Data misrep-resentation; undisclosed conflict of interest	Profound global impact on public health policy and publication ethics
2002	Jan Hendrik Schön case	Data fabrication	Highlighted importance of raw data preservation and independent verification
2004–2006	Hwang Woo-Suk stem cell fraud	Fabrication in biomedical research	Led to reforms in peer review scrutiny and ethical oversight
2010–2012	Anil Potti investigation (India)	Translational research falsification	Emphasized need for data transparency and reproducibility

Year	Event	Nature of Misconduct	Regulatory Impact
2011	Diederik Stapel case	Fabricated social science data	Raised concerns on research culture, mentorship, and academic pressure
2012	Yoshitaka Fujii case	Mass fabricated clinical trials	Strengthened statistical screening in journals
2014–2018	Paolo Macchiarini case	Misrepresent-ed surgical outcomes	Highlighted link between publication ethics and patient safety
2018	UGC Plagiarism Regulations (India)	Academic plagiarism control	Mandatory similarity screening in universities
2021–2023	Large-scale Paper Mill Investigations	Organized manuscript fabrication	Strengthened publisher policies, authorship verification, and screening processes

Chapter 6

Databases and Research Metrics

Dr. Rajesh Kumar Gandhirajan
Professor, Dept of Human Genetics, FBMST
Rajesh.gandhirajan@sriramachandra.edu.in

Abstract:

Due to current advances in digital databases and quantitative measures that are affecting the discovery, evaluation, and dissemination of research, it is necessary for researchers to understand these systems and their implications when conducting their own research and publishing ethically. This chapter provides an overview of scholarly databases (e.g., Web of Science, Scopus) in the research ecosystem and discusses indexing vs. citation databases and their role in organization and tracking of scholarly literature. It includes a discussion of coverage, selection criteria, and analytic functions from major citation databases such as Web of Science and Scopus. The chapter examines journal-level metrics (e.g., Journal Impact Factor, Cite Score, SNIP, SJR, and IPP) as well as author-level metrics (e.g., h-index, g-index, and i10-index). Additionally, the chapter includes an examination of alternative indicators or altimetric that measure engagement with research in non-traditional ways or across societal domains such as academia and community engagement. Lastly, the chapter discusses ethical issues associated with using metrics to evaluate research and explores several international initiatives focused on promoting the use of responsible metrics in evaluating research. The chapter seeks to equip researchers with the conceptual skills necessary for the critical interpretation and responsible utilization of research measures by merging technical explanations with ethical considerations.

Learning Objectives:

After Completing the chapter, the reader will be able to

- Explain the role of scholarly databases in organizing, discovering, and accessing academic literature within the global research ecosystem.
- Identify major international and national research databases and understand their inclusion criteria and coverage.
- Describe the concept of research metrics and explain how bibliometric indicators are used to measure scholarly productivity and influence.
- Recognize ethical concerns related to the misuse of research metrics, including metric manipulation, citation cartels, and predatory publishing practices.

1. Introduction:

In recent decades there has been a significant and rapid increase in the amount of scientific research published globally, which has changed how scholarly knowledge is organized, accessed, and evaluated. The way that academics communicate with each other has developed into an infrastructure using digital technology and has included indexing platforms, citation databases, and quantitative metrics of academic performance.

In addition to assisting with discovering new information, databases and research metrics play an ever-increasingly important role in academic careers, institutional decision-making, and funding priorities for research.

The introduction of citation indexing during the latter half of the 20th century brought about major changes to the organization of scholarly literature. By linking publications to each other through citations, citation indexing provided a means for tracking intellectual influence across different disciplines and over time. Eugene Garfield's original research established the theoretical foundation for today's citation databases to be created as rigorous tools for measuring the flow of intellectual information. The systems of citation indexing have changed since then to more than just indexing publications; the additional features added provided ways to analyse data from publications, authorship collaboration patterns, and trends in citation rates.

Currently, in today's world, both Scopus and Web of Science are the largest libraries of bibliographic information. The basis of contemporary bibliometric studies is primarily built on citation identification algorithms, how journals are chosen, and the structure of bibliographical information about the articles. Being included in these databases greatly influences the visibility of research. If a piece of research is not included in these databases, there is a much greater likelihood that it will not be found or cited. In this regard, the inclusion or exclusion of a database can have evaluative consequences rather than merely technical ones.

The creation of metrics used to evaluate research has been done in conjunction with the appearance of the first citation databases. The Journal Impact Factor, Cite Score, h-index, etc., originally served as tools to assist librarians with managing their collections by identifying citation patterns. However, the use of these metrics has slowly changed to more of an evaluative nature. Internet publications will line up their recruiting, promotion, funding distribution, and ranking decisions according to quantitative measures more often than not in many academic environments today. Therefore, there is a substantial relationship between practical value and ethical discussions pertaining to the changes made in the use of quantitative metrics versus descriptive statistics.

While the use of metrics may provide some degree of efficiency and comparability in research publication because of the large volumes of article submissions being submitted, there are also some displacements. Each discipline, type of publication (i.e., book, journal article, conference paper, etc.), and each stage in an individual's career will show significant differences in citation practices. A numerical indicator may elevate certain disciplines, publication language, and forms of collaboration over others. The use of metrical values in evaluating scholarship will not capture the entirety of a complicated scholarly contribution if the metric's context is not understood.

Therefore, understanding the various databases and their associated metrics is a necessary aspect of research and publication ethics. Using these systems ethically requires more than just basic technical understanding of the databases; it also requires knowledge regarding the methodologies upon which they are based, their limitations, and the degree to which they can be applied. This chapter outlines the structure and functions of indexing and citations databases, evaluates various metrics of total publications (the total number of articles published in a journal) and authorship (the number of authors on an individual article), and considers emerging alternative metrics of the visibility of scholarly research. In addition, the chapter outlines the ethical principles used to guide the evaluation of scholarly research and the balance that must exist between quantitative and qualitative evaluations of research.

With the current emphasis on quantifying the impact of scholarship, it is necessary for anyone using scholarly metrics to have a basic understanding of how to read and evaluate metrics in a way that ensures fairness, transparency, and integrity in the academic world.

2. Scholarly Databases:

Scholarly databases are the main form of the digital infrastructure for organizing, discovering and accessing academic knowledge. The sheer amount of scientific literature produced in so many fields has led to the scholarly database becoming an essential tool for researchers, librarians, and institutions to find relevant research and assess the amount of scholarly work being produced. Instead of just being a way to store documents, scholarly databases are structured information systems that use standardized metadata; controlled vocabularies; and indexing protocols to catalogue (put into a system of categories) publications.

Scholarly databases share two important purposes that are connected with each other. First, they provide a systematic way to discover research by organizing literature by subject category, author, Institution and publication details. Second, they provide an avenue for the analysis of scholarly communication principles through citation relationships and other bibliography-based metadata linking to the publication. Through the combination of both functions, through the use of cited works, researchers can trace the development of scientific ideas, find out the most important works, and evaluate patterns of research activity.

One of the main ways scholarly databases differ from other databases is the way the content contained in them is decided upon through a specific set of requirements that each source of publication must meet before being included. To be published in a journal, most journals and other sources of publication would require a standard academic peer-review process, an editorial review, consistency in publication, and honesty in reporting the content submitted for publication. These criteria differentiate academic databases from general web search engines, which typically include content automatically and without filters. Thus, journalism content found in a database implies that the journal has met some minimum criteria for being legitimate, but being included in a database does not necessarily mean that every individual article included will also be scientifically high quality.

Classification of Scholarly Databases:

Academic databases can generally be divided into two major types according to their primary function: indexing and citation databases. Both types of academic databases aid researchers in finding research, but each has its own particular type of information and its own type of tools for helping researchers to access research on the web. Knowing the difference between indexing databases and citation databases is critical for understanding how visible research is, what the journal's claims are for being indexed by various databases, and how to use bibliometric data that comes from different databases of citations.

Indexing databases serve primarily as bibliographic catalogues of scholarly publications that are arranged by topic, by keyword, by author, and by publication source. The primary purpose of an indexing database is to enhance the ability to find research literature, and each indexing database generally will list the journals and articles in a systematic manner through a structured system of classification. In indexing databases, the records typically contain items that have bibliographic metadata such as the article title, abstract, author name, institutional affiliation, and keywords; however, indexing databases do not generally provide any information about the citation relationships between publications.

Indexing databases typically require journals to meet certain standards through an evaluation process. This evaluation may include evaluating if the journal is peer-reviewed, if it has a valid editorial board, if it publishes transparently, and if it follows publication ethics. As a result of this screening process, many research institutions and regulatory agencies rely on indexing status as an initial evaluation of whether or not a journal is credible.

Examples of major indexing databases include MEDLINE, a comprehensive index of biomedical literature; the Directory of Open Access Journals (DOAJ) for high-quality open-access journals; Chemical Abstracts Service (CAS), which is a comprehensive indexing service covering chemicals and molecular research; and UGC-CARE, an Indian database designed to assist researchers with finding reputable publication outlets.

While indexing helps researchers find and categorize scholarly literature, it has limitations. Indexing databases provide access to scholarly literature; however, they do not evaluate the quality of research or the number of times the research has been cited. Therefore, an index status should not be assumed as a direct reflection of research impact.

Citation databases build on the functionality of indexing databases by systematically recording the citation links that exist between scholarly publications. These citation links are the references that are cited in articles, and they form connections that exist between research outputs across time and across disciplines. Citation tracking allows researchers to examine how the development of an idea has evolved over time, which pieces of research have influenced later research, and how the scholarly community interacts through referencing research.

Prominent examples of citation databases include Web of Science and Scopus. These platforms index not only journals, but also perform analyses on the relationships between citations to provide an array of bibliometric indicators, which can be used for research evaluation. Citation databases provide the structure for calculating and presenting a variety of metrics, including journal impact indicators, author indices, and performance indicators for institutions based on their research output.

Unlike indexing databases, citation databases offer researchers access to analytical tools that solidly enable researchers to identify citation networks, track trends in research, and assess the scholarly influence of research. However, indexing databases and citation databases do not share the same coverage with respect to disciplinary representation, journal inclusion policies, and geographical diversity. Therefore, when utilizing citation-based information for analysis, users must be aware of the scope of the citation database they are using and the limitations that apply to all citation database citations.

Indexes serve two different purposes as indexing and citation databases, although sometimes being referred to interchangeably. The indexing databases are designed to help you discover new or additional scholarly literature by organising, cataloguing, and indexing it. Citation databases, however, are designed to assist you in the discovery of scholarly literature, as well as tracking how publications reference one another, thus allowing you to assess the impact of research and the influence of scholars.

By understanding the difference between indexing and citation databases, you can accurately interpret what claims there are regarding whether or not a journal is indexed, you will also be able to assess the research metrics associated with research activity, and you can more clearly grasp the overall structure of research communication.

3. Research Metrics:

Through the creation of citation databases, scholars now have the ability to positively discover the literature available to them and quantitatively analyse the research activity. The citation databases provide quantifiable information by collecting and recording all citation relationships between publications, thus creating large data sets that can assist in identifying the patterns of communication among scholars. The patterns identified lead to the development of research metrics, which are numerical values used to help summarize the extent to which researchers are productive, the extent to which they influence other researchers, and how much they disseminate research.

Research metrics were originally intended to support librarians and information professionals in understanding the citation behaviour of scholars, as well as managing journal collections. The role of research metrics is very expanded; however, it continues to have a major role within the academic system. It has become common practice for universities, governmental funding agencies, and regulating organizations to utilize metric-based indicators to provide guidance for decisions relating to hiring, promotion, funding distribution, and rank at an institution. Although metric-based indicators can provide a quick summary of large amounts of publication data, there are limitations to using such indicators solely among themselves. The numerical values found on these indicators may not reflect the entire intellectual quality or societal contribution of any given research study.

Research metrics can be broken down into three categories: journal-level metrics, author-level metrics, and article-level metrics. The specific use of research metrics is usually dependent upon which type of research metric is being utilized to evaluate the study in question. Therefore, in order for research metrics to be used appropriately in the assessment of research, it is necessary to understand their methodological basis and the limitations each type of metric has.

Journal-level Metrics:

Journal metrics measure how many times research is cited, with the citation counts measuring academic journals rather than individual research articles or all researchers affiliated with those journals. The way in which journal-level metrics are measured is a summary of how many times the articles published in a specific journal have been cited during a predetermined period. Originally, journalist metrics were used to compare journals only within the same subject area; however, many researchers use these metrics as benchmarks for the perceived quality of research published in those journals, which is not the intent of these metrics.

The Journal Impact Factor (JIF), which is computed annually using data from the Journal Citation Reports (JCR) database developed by Clarivate Analytics, is one of the best-known journal impact factors. Average citations per published document.

The Average Cite Rate (Cite Score) at least gives you an idea of what the average journal article is cited at and has been compared to Cite Factor (IF) as a measure of success, with the same definition for both, however other metrics have used different time spans and included different types of documents.

In the context of journals there have been many attempts to develop metrics that use citation counts adjusted for a variety of reasons including differing norms across disciplines and the different types of documents that could be counted as published articles in a journal. With the creation of new journals, particularly those published on the Internet, many of these same metrics have now been developed or are being developed for those journals. However, they have not all been uniformly defined or reported because of the wide variety of alternate metrics being created and reported. One metric that has been developed is Source Normalized Impact per Paper (SNIP) which attempts to normalize/re-weight citation counts based on typical citation behaviour within specific disciplines to enable researchers to make more accurate comparisons between disciplines.

Source Normalized Impact per Paper (SNIP) provides average citation counts for a specific document type (i.e., journal article) within a specific journal's citation distribution (i.e., normalizing citation counts across time) in addition to providing comparisons to other document types from other journals in other disciplines.

The Citation Index is a useful indicator of the impact of an article in the world of academic publishing because consistent usage of the same criteria for determining the total breadth of article citations received within an author's research discipline enables researchers to examine the overall impact of both the journal and specific articles included in the journal relative to each other. The SCImago Journal Rank (SJR) uses a prestige-based methodology for measuring citation influence from different sources within the citation networks. The SJR weight places more importance on citations from higher-ranked journals compared to those from lower-ranked journals. The Impact per Publication (IPP) is also considered when determining the average number of times an article in a journal has been cited within three years of being published, and IPP serves as a basis for calculating SNIP.

Even though the methodologies for calculating these metrics are very different, they all share the same characteristic of describing citation patterns at the journal level only as opposed to measuring the impact of individual articles. Therefore, many scholars warn against using journal metrics as direct measures of research quality.

Author-level Metrics:

Bibliometrics generally focus on the publication venue where the research is published; however, bibliometrics at the author level attempt to measure the impact of individual researchers. These bibliometric indicators are generally based on the citation performance of a researcher's publications in the leading bibliometric databases (Web of Science, Scopus, and Google Scholar).

The h-index developed by physicist Jorge E. Hirsch in 2005 is one of the most frequently used author-level bibliometric indicators. An author is said to have an h-index if they have publications that have received at least h citations. The "h-index" merges two parts of a scholar's performance - their output (which is published work) and their influence (a count of how well this work has been cited). Its combination of an output-based metric (productivity) with an impact-based metric (impact) has made it one of the more popular means for evaluating scholarly work in research.

However, there are also some fundamental weaknesses associated with the h-index. The h-index generally increases with time in academia; therefore, it tends to disadvantage early-career scholars relative to established researchers. In addition, the h-index does not take into account differences in citation practices across disciplines, nor does it consider cases where multiple authors contribute to a scholarly project, resulting in collaborative research.

To try and overcome some of the shortcomings of the h-index, other types of author-level measures have been suggested. For instance, the g-index, developed by Leo Egghe, offers additional weight to those works that have been significantly cited, based on the cumulative citation counts of the most influential articles published by a given author. The i10-index, which counts the number of times an author's article has been cited at least ten times, is also a commonly used author-level metric. The i10-index is readily available to use via an individual's Google Scholar profile and provides an immediate picture of that author's citation activity.

Author-level metrics are useful references for determining an individual's volume of work and productivity in terms of scholarly output; however, when using these measures in making conclusions as to the author's standing, it is also important to understand the context in which the work was produced, as disciplinary and career stage factors are influential in determining an author's citation count.

Article-level Metrics:

In contrast to the journal or author metrics, article level metrics indicate the impact (performance) of an individual piece of research. For example, you can use article level metrics such as the number of citations; download statistics; usage metrics related to a specific document (e.g. URL usage data); etc. to evaluate the impact of an individual research article. Article-level metrics allow researchers and evaluators to assess the influence of one individual research article instead of relying on the reputation of the journal or on aggregate author statistics.

The number of citations is still the most popular article-level metric and can be found in a variety of citation databases, such as the Web of Science, Scopus, and Google Scholar. Although citations often take a long time to accumulate (nut longer than it takes to get published) (more so for publication types that tend to have longer publication cycles), other ways to measure article-level impact could be through the number of times an article is downloaded, viewed, referenced, or engaged with by someone online.

Altmetrics:

Because of the rise of the use of digital communication platforms/ technologies, there has been an increase in attention paid to alternative metrics (often referred to as altmetrics). These are indicators of the online engagement (or the wider participation) with that piece of research, such as when references to that research appear on social media (e.g. Facebook and Twitter), when that research gets covered by a news organisation and when it is referenced in Government policy documents (e.g. legislation and policy documents), and when it is stored in an online reference manager (e.g. Mendeley).

The composite measures of various articles including these create an overall composite measure of the digital visibility of a research article and are often consolidated in databases such as Altmetric and PlumX to provide insight into the overall digital visibility of a specific article. Unlike traditional citation metrics, which merely cover academic reputation, altmetrics provide information on how scholarship is shared and talked about within a wider audience or professional community.

On the other hand, while altmetrics are excellent at showing very quick responses to research, they have several challenges. Engagement online can be the result of promotional efforts to increase content visibility, how social media is used by users, and how bots artificially boost content visibility, all of which may not provide indications of scientific quality. For this reason, altmetrics should be considered as complementary metrics that give additional context to scholarship and should not replace traditional bibliometric measures.

Research metrics are valuable tools for summarising scholarly productivity, but in order to properly interpret them, they must be put into contextual perspective. For example, citation practices differ considerably among areas of research, publication types and types of researchers. Therefore, numerical indicators may reflect the process of scholarly communication rather than providing an indication of the research itself. Understanding then limitations of metrics is critical to ensure that scholarly activity is evaluated judiciously, rather than simply relying on expert opinion.

4. Ethical Use and Misuse of Databases and Research Metrics:

There has been a significant shift in how academic institutions assess research performance because of the increased use of scholarly databases and quantitative measures. These tools allow researchers to efficiently organize and source the massive quantity of scholarly content generated today, but their use in assessing research performance raises a number of ethical issues. If databases and metrics are interpreted without understanding their contextual impacts, they can hinder academic priorities, incentivize superficial methods of measurement, and detract from the overall goals of scientific research.

One of the most pressing ethical issues involves using journal-level measures to evaluate individual research output. The Journal Impact Factor (JIF) was originally developed to assess citation patterns across journals and to assist libraries with managing journal subscriptions. However, they ultimately have come to be used as a substitute measure of the quality of a researcher's work or a researcher's competency rather than as a tool for assessing how well a researcher has performed in their discipline. Such uses oversimplify the scholarly assessment process because citation patterns differ dramatically depending on the discipline, research topic, and type of publication. For example, the most frequently cited articles published in large-volume journals frequently will not have been published in journals with high-impact factors, nor will they have been published in large-volume journals compared with the most highly cited articles published in lower-volume journals.

Another significant ethical challenge exists with the rise of metric-driven academic environments. In these environments, the primary focus is on the number of publications produced by a researcher, thus making it difficult to distinguish between success as a researcher and other variables that are influencing success.

The emergence of metric-driven academic cultures (especially since the publication count and citation count have become the primary means of measuring success) creates another challenge for researchers because their opportunity for advancement is determined significantly by numerical measures. This can lead researchers to feel pressured to employ strategies that will yield quantifiable outputs rather than focusing on scientific integrity. The pressure created by the necessity for researchers to produce quantifiable outputs can allow researchers to engage in unethical practices such as self-citation, citation cartels, and arranging author contributions strategically to increase the likelihood of receiving citations.

Additionally, the misuse of databases and metrics has contributed to the increase in predatory publishing. Predatory journals take advantage of researchers having incomplete knowledge or understanding of the criteria by which journals are indexed in a database and use this misunderstanding of criteria to present themselves as legitimate journals (e.g., by making false claims about being indexed in particular databases or claiming fictitious impact factors) although these journals typically do not have a rigorous peer review or editorial policy in place. Researchers may unintentionally submit their work to these predatory journals because of institutional pressure to produce a certain number of publications; therefore, these researchers jeopardize the integrity of their research and their academic integrity.

Creating a more responsible method of evaluating research is the solution to these challenges; several international initiatives have developed to promote the ethical use of metrics in research evaluation. Two important frameworks that guide researchers as they think about research and metrics in evaluating research output are the San Francisco Declaration on Research Assessment (DORA) and The Leiden Manifesto. The focus of DORA is that metrics related to journals should not be used to evaluate either the quality of particular individual articles or the quality of researchers. The Declaration instead encourages institutions to consider that research outputs have intrinsic merit and that many forms of scholarly impact should be considered in evaluating research.

Likewise, the Leiden Manifesto consists of guiding principles for research metrics to be used responsibly. Key recommendations include that the use of quantitative indicators should supplement but not replace using expert assessment, that evaluation practices should take into account the differences between disciplines when it comes to citation behavior, and that the data used in calculating metrics should be both transparent and able to be verified. The manifesto warns against the false sense of precision that numerical rankings give to researchers, as there are many aspects of a scholar's contribution to research that cannot be captured by a single score.

In order for researchers, administrators and evaluators to interact ethically with databases and research metrics, there needs to be a level of metric literacy developed. The more researchers, administrators and evaluators know about how databases identify journals, how citation indicators are developed, and the limitations of those measures, the more balanced and knowledgeable they will be when interpreting metrics. While metrics may aid in revealing trends related to scholarly communications, they should not be regarded as absolute measures of the quality of research.

The role of metrics as tools is to aid in revealing patterns in scholarly communications (e.g., bibliometrics) while recognizing both their value and limitations. For responsible assessment of research in the context of Research and Publication Ethics, there needs to be a balance between using quantitative metrics and using qualitative methods for assessing academic work. By being mindful of both the strengths and weaknesses of these tools, and continuously striving to use them appropriately, the academic community will ultimately support transparency and accountability, without compromising the core values essential to successful scientific endeavours.

5. Conclusion:

Due to the rapid increase in scholarly literature, it is necessary to have systems that can organise, retrieve, and assess research products at the global level; thus, a system has been developed to be able to allow scientists to evaluate and find vast amounts of research, as well as recognise and evaluate how they have impacted each other. Finding research through indexed databases allows for systematic cataloguing of research and research products (academic publications), which allows for the improvement of the discoverability of research. Finding research through citation databases allows for a systematic cataloguing of relationships between research and how authors are impacted by the citations of their works. When combined, indexed databases and citation databases provide the foundation of data for bibliometric studies conducted by scientists.

Research metrics that have been developed from indexed and citation databases offer a means to summarise the publication and citation history of research. Through the use of journal metrics, author indices, emerging article level and alternative metrics, scientists can analyse the results of research within the academic and public domains. Nonetheless, the current trend to heavily rely on research metrics has also shed light on their weaknesses. Because citation patterns differ between disciplines, publication types and stages of a researcher's career, alone using only a numerical or statistically based system does not provide a complete depiction of innovative, rigorous and/or valuable research to society.

To ethically evaluate research, we require a variety of types of evaluation; quantitative indicators to supplement the expert opinions of your peers. The ethical frameworks of research assessment (like the San Francisco Declaration on Research Assessment and the Leiden Manifesto) make it clear that research assessment should acknowledge the content and contribution of all forms of scholarly research rather than relying on journal or citation based indicators alone.

In today's increasingly data-driven academic environment, researchers must develop an understanding of how databases and metrics work, how they measure data, and how to distinguish between what they measure and what they do not measure. If used judiciously and interpreted appropriately and in the context of the applicable discipline, data and metrics will provide greater transparency and inform scholarly assessment than they would if used uncritically; however, if used without consideration of their validity they may limit the full understanding of a scholarly product's impact and may spur metric-driven behavior. The ethical use of data and research metrics is critical to developing a fair and respectful global community of scholars, integrity in scholarship and intellectual diversity in the global scholarly community.

References:

1. Yadav, S. K. (2023). Database and research metrics. In *Research and Publication Ethics* (pp. 229-250). Cham: Springer International Publishing.

2. Eltaybani, S., Lange, J., & Golla, M. (2025). Research Metrics: An Overview. *AJN The American Journal of Nursing, 125*(10), 61-63.

3. Wanyama, S. B., McQuaid, R. W., & Kittler, M. (2022). Where you search determines what you find: the effects of bibliographic databases on systematic reviews. *International journal of social research methodology, 25*(3), 409-422.

4. Ivanović, L., Baaden, P., Jovanović, M., & Ivanović, D. (2025). Correlation between journal metrics-based academic evaluation and researchers' ethics. *Accountability in research, 32*(4), 459-487.

5. Koerber, A., Starkey, J., Ardon-Dryer, K., Cummins, R. G., Eko, L., & Kee, K. (2023). *The predatory paradox: Ethics, politics, and practices in contemporary scholarly publishing* (p. 284). Open Book Publishers.

Chapter 7

Composition and Functions of Institutional Ethics Committees

Dr. Aruna Subramaniam, PhD in Nursing
Professor and HOD,
Sri Ramachandra Faculty of Nursing, SRIHER(DU)
Mail id : aruna.s@sriramachandra.edu.in

Learning Objectives for this Chapter:

After reading this chapter, the reader will be able to:

1. Explain the purpose and importance of Institutional Ethics Committees (IECs) in protecting human participants in research.

2. Describe the composition and multidisciplinary membership of an Ethics Committee according to national and international guidelines.

3. Identify the roles and responsibilities of various IEC members involved in ethical review.

4. Discuss the functions and ethical review processes followed by IECs for research involving human participants.

5. Understand the ethical principles and regulatory requirements guiding research oversight and participant protection.

Abstract:

This chapter investigates the composition and the role of Institutional Ethics Committees (IECs) in the context of the Standards and Operational Guidance for Ethics Review of Health-Related Research with Human Participants from the World Health Organization (WHO, 2011), and the National Ethical Guidelines for Biomedical and Health Research Involving Human Participants from the Indian Council of Medical Research (ICMR, 2017). It describes the organizational and procedural standards to create a reliable research ethics review system. The standards emphasize institutional accountability, independence, appropriate resources, and transparency. The chapter examines the multidisciplinary nature of the membership of IECs and the minimum number of members required to make decisions about ethics review. The chapter also explores the representation of medical, legal, social, and community members in IECs to provide a balanced consideration during ethics deliberation. Furthermore, the chapter examines the specific decision-making criteria in the area of ethics, which include scientific validity, risk-benefit analysis, participant selection, obtaining informed consent, protecting confidentiality, and considering community impacts. In addition to ethics decision-making criteria, the chapter provides an overview of administrative responsibilities of IECs, the importance of creating written standard operating procedures, documentation, and continuous monitoring and evaluation mechanisms. The chapter also addresses the obligations of researchers in securing approval, reporting safety problems, and complying with regulations. Overall, the standards outlined in this chapter emphasize accountability for participants' protection and ethics integrity in biomedical and health research conducted with human participants.

Keywords:

Institutional Ethics Committee; Ethical Review System; Human Participant Protection; Research Governance; Informed Consent; Regulatory Compliance

Introduction:

Ethics Committees (ECs) are essential to protect the dignity, rights, safety and welfare of participants in research. Prior to initiating any health research using human subjects, biological samples or data (clinical research, basic science research, and behavioural research), researchers must obtain prior approval from their EC. The institution hosting the researcher bears the responsibility for developing and implementing an effective, long-term review system for research and for supporting its logistics, which include funding, physical space, and time for the Member Secretary. An EC must be able to conduct both scientific and ethical assessments of proposed research, and it must continuously monitor the research it has approved to ensure that it remains ethically compliant.

Standard 1: Accountability for Developing the Research Ethics Review System:

National and institutional authorities have the primary responsibility for developing and maintaining a viable and efficient system for the ethical review of health-related research involving human participants. This involves developing a comprehensive legislative and regulatory framework based upon internationally recognised ethical principles. Within this framework, national and institutional authorities must establish competent and independent Ethics Committees (ECs) at the national, regional, and/or institutional levels, and across both public and private sectors. National and institutional authorities must also establish stable mechanisms to evaluate and improve the quality, uniformity, and effectiveness of the ethical review process on a periodic basis. While there is considerable focus on how individual ECs perform, they are unable to perform effectively without the broader framework of a human research protection system. A systems-based approach ensures that ethical oversight is coordinated and consistent, and that it receives adequate support at various levels of governance.

All research involving human subjects should normally be reviewed by an EC. Ethical oversight is expected to occur in virtually all cases of research involving human participants. However, there are some types of research that involve minimal risks that may be exempted from full review or eligible for expedited review, provided exemptions and expedited reviews are permitted under national regulations and align with internationally accepted ethical standards.

Furthermore, ECs should serve as key elements of a larger research participant protection program. The larger framework would include structured education programs for EC members and investigators, as well as systems to increase efficiency, accountability, and consistency in review procedures. National governments will be responsible for directing, coordinating, and supporting these systems to maintain public trust and to foster ethics integrity. In addition to promoting cooperation among ECs operating at the institutional, regional, and national levels, well-established processes should exist to facilitate effective communication and collaboration among them. Such cooperation could take the form of standardising procedures, facilitating networking among professionals, and granting access to decisions previously made regarding ethics review. Such coordination is particularly important in the case of multi-centre and multi-national research, where streamlined and non-repetitive review processes are needed.

The ethics review system must also be coordinated with national regulatory agencies responsible for overseeing pharmaceuticals, biologics, and medical devices. Coordination with national and international clinical trial registries would also contribute to increased transparency and compliance with regulations.

Additionally, mechanisms should be developed to integrate community viewpoints into the ethics review process. Community participation in the ethics review process can help institutions respond to local culture, social contexts, and concerns of participants.

Finally, a formal registry of ECs operating within a nation should be created and maintained. Registry development increases transparency, facilitates oversight, and promotes compliance with established ethics standards.

Types of Research Reviewed by ECs:

Ethics committees are responsible for the review of a wide variety of research designs and methodologies. Examples of research designs and methodologies include clinical trials to evaluate the efficacy of treatments or prevention methods, epidemiologic studies to identify and characterize the distribution and causes of disease, social/behavioural research; studies using identifiable patient (or other) information from medical records; research involving stored biological samples;

health system research; and implementation research focused on improving healthcare delivery

In light of this variety in research methodology, ECs will require knowledge of many different scientific methods and the associated ethical concerns that arise with each method of science. This knowledge of research designs, data management practices, privacy protections, risks assessments, and context-specific ethical considerations will be required for making informed, balanced, and ethical decisions regarding a research protocol.

Standard 2: Composition of research ethics committees:

The structure of a Research Ethics Committee (REC) is designed to promote independence, credibility, and balanced decision making in assessing the ethical merit of research studies conducted on humans. A REC that reflects diversity in professional backgrounds, industry/sector representations, and gender/age will provide a high-quality and diverse array of viewpoints in its assessment of proposed research projects.

A REC must be composed of multiple discipline and multi-sector representatives. For example, the REC could consist of physicians, biologists, lawyers, sociologists, ethicists, and representatives of various sectors, which would help to prevent narrow/biased assessments of proposed research and would promote a comprehensive assessment of each project.

Age and gender diversity among committee members is equally as important as diversity among disciplines and sectors; these elements provide for richer and more sensitive discussions regarding the needs of various participant groups. In addition, there may be instances where gender-balancing is critical (e.g., studies involving women, children or other vulnerable populations).

In order to ensure the independence of the REC from the institution conducting the research, it is recommended that at least 50% of the members have no affiliation with the institution. Members having no affiliation with the institution, i.e., members who are not employed by the institution, provide a level of objectivity to the assessment process and increase public confidence in the validity of the committees' decisions.

The number of members on the REC typically ranges from 7 to 15. While this provides sufficient expertise for evaluating research proposals, it maintains a level of operational efficiency for the committee. In order for a meeting to occur and officially conduct business, a quorum of at least 5 members must be present. If fewer than 5 members are present at the time of the meeting, no decisions made during the meeting are considered valid.

In terms of balance within the committee, the REC should reflect a mix of medical and non-medical members, as well as technical and non-technical members. For example, medical members are those who possess the proper medical credentials to assess the medical implications of proposed research studies, whereas technical members are those who possess the necessary knowledge/experience to assess the technical merit of proposed research studies (for example, sociologists). These levels of balance are based on the institution's research profile, however, must always be representative of all components of the research study.

Roles, Affiliations, Qualifications, and Responsibilities of EC Members:

The effectiveness of the EC is dependent upon the clear roles and responsibilities of the EC members as well as their composition.

The Chairperson and if available the Vice Chairperson of the EC must be non-affiliated to provide independence to the EC. The ideal candidate would be someone with a high level of respect from the academic community from any professional background with past experience serving on an ethics committee. The Chairperson will lead the meetings and be accountable for the effective and unbiased functioning of the EC. All members especially the non-affiliated and non-clinical members of the EC should participate actively in the discussion and decision-making processes. The Chairperson will approve the minutes of past meetings and ensure that the EC's decision-making process is transparent. If neither the Chairperson nor the Vice Chairperson are able to attend a meeting, the EC can nominate an Acting Chairperson (who must be non-affiliated) prior to the meeting or elect one through a vote of the members attending the meeting. The Acting Chairperson will have full authority for the duration of the meeting. The Chairperson is also responsible for requesting declarations of potential conflicts of interest from EC members, assuring that the quorum is met, promoting fair decision making and resolving complaints regarding researchers, EC members, conflicts of interest or requests for access to EC documents.

The Member Secretary and when needed the Alternate Member Secretary must be affiliated with the institution. Ideally the Member Secretary would be an administrative employee of the institution with prior experience and knowledge of clinical research and ethics and good communication skills. The Member Secretary is responsible for organizing and coordinating the entire review process. Duties of the Member Secretary include receiving research proposals, determining whether the documentation received is complete, drafting and distributing agendas, arranging for meetings, keeping records and archives of the EC's deliberations and decisions and recording the minutes of the deliberations and decisions. The Member Secretary is also responsible for updating the standard operating procedures (SOPs) and following them strictly; arranging training for the EC members and the administrative personnel supporting the EC; and preparing for audits or inspections. The Member Secretary will determine whether a proposal is exempt from review, eligible for expedited review or requires full review, and determine if a prior scientific review or consultation with independent experts or community representatives is required. The institution must also protect sufficient time for the Member Secretary to adequately perform the tasks outlined above.

Basic Medical Scientist members can be affiliated or unaffiliated members of the EC. Basic Medical Scientist members must have either medical or non-medical qualifications in basic medical sciences. In the case of clinical trials that involve drugs, it is preferred that the Basic Medical Scientist be a pharmacologist. Their primary role is to conduct a scientific and ethical evaluation of the research proposals submitted to the EC, focusing on such items as the specifics of the interventions, the risks versus benefits associated with the proposed research, the research design, the methodology used to collect data, the statistical validity of the study and the continued review process. The Basic Medical Scientist will also evaluate Serious Adverse Event Reports.

protocol deviations, progress updates, and completion reports. In drug trials, the pharmacologist evaluates drug safety and pharmacodynamics to ensure participant protection.

Healthcare professionals/ **Clinicians,** involved with the oversight of a study, either as affiliated personnel or unaffiliated individuals, are required to have professional medical qualifications and appropriate experience/training relative to their role on the study. The healthcare professionals' responsibilities include, but are not limited to, reviewing the clinical aspects of the protocol; determining the appropriateness of the intervention(s) proposed; evaluating the risk-benefit ratio associated with each intervention; reviewing the study's methodology; verifying that an adequate number of subjects is included in the study population; ensuring that the location(s) selected for the study are suitable for conducting the study; reviewing and evaluating the study's statistical considerations; reviewing the status of ongoing studies to which they have provided approval (including, but not limited to, review of Serious Adverse Events (SAEs), Protocol Violations, Periodic Progress Reports); determining whether adequate medical facilities are available at each study site; determining the competency of investigators conducting the study; and reviewing the plans for providing medical care for those subjects injured during the course of the study, and the mechanism by which compensation will be made available to such subjects. As part of this responsibility, the healthcare professionals will thoroughly evaluate each document submitted in support of the application, including, but not limited to, the Investigator Brochure when applicable.

Legal experts, which may include both affiliated and non-affiliated members, is comprised of lawyers that have a law degree from a reputable law school and preferably have some background in legal practice and are trained in Medical Law. These lawyers will review all Informed Consent Documents (ICDs) and translations, Memorandums of Understanding (MoUs), Clinical Trial Agreements (CTAs), regulatory approvals, insurance documents, site permissions, and researcher undertakings. The lawyers will determine whether the above items comply with local regulations and specific approval requirements (e.g., stem cell research, international collaborations). The legal expert on the committee will also advise the committee of any new regulations or changes to existing laws.

A social scientist, philosopher, ethicist, or theologian may serve as either an affiliated or non-affiliated member. He/she is expected to have academic background in the social and behavioral sciences; in philosophy; or in religious studies; and be sensitive to local cultural and moral beliefs. Such Members can be affiliated with non-governmental organizations that are involved in health-related issues. The Member will review research proposals and informed consent forms, assess potential impacts on communities, and evaluate the implications of research findings from socio-cultural, religious or philosophical aspects. As a representative of both the society and the participant, he/she will raise larger ethical concerns when they arise.

Lay persons Involving community members in the process of reviewing the ethics of research on their community allows for input by people who are representative of that community. These individuals would ideally be active in the community, know the local culture and language, and have some familiarity with the community's values and traditions. Non-professional reviewers would provide an assessment of how clearly and easily understandable the information being provided to participants was; whether the potential benefits of participation outweighed the possible risks; and identify any potential issues that might arise as a result of the research (e.g., harm to future generations).

Quorum Requirements:

The IEC must have a minimum number of members present for each meeting to be legally and procedurally valid according to regulatory guidelines provided by the Central Drugs Standard Control Organisation (CDSCO). As such, there are at least 5 members that must be physically present when reviewing each research protocol. In addition to providing a balanced view of expertise, these individuals must also provide a variety of perspectives to allow for complete ethical analysis. The required participation is as follows: A basic medical scientist — preferably a pharmacologist — to examine the scientific and pharmacological aspects of the study; a clinician to assess the clinical significance of the trial and the safety of participants; a legal representative to assess whether the trial complies with all relevant laws and regulations; a social scientist or an individual representing a non-governmental, voluntary organisation, philosopher, ethicist, theologian or similar professional to assess the social-ethics of the trial; and a layperson from the community to assess the public interest and protect the rights of the participants.

In addition to being comprised of professionals with diverse backgrounds and areas of expertise, the quorum must include both medical and non-medical members to provide both technical and non-technical perspectives on the issue at hand. Ideally, it would be desirable to have at least one member who does not work for the institution, to preserve impartiality and prevent bias towards the institution. Ideally, a layperson should be included in the quorum to reflect the views of the community. Regulatory clinical trials require that the quorum meet CDSCO's current requirements. Any decisions made at meetings where the required number of members were not present, or did not have the necessary expertise and/or representation will be deemed invalid and therefore not be regarded as an official decision of the Ethics Committee.

Additional Provisions:

The Head of the Institution should not be a member of the EC in order to maintain the independence of the EC. The Head may however act as an Appellate Authority and make decisions regarding appointments to committees or resolve disputes.

The Chairperson and the Member Secretary may hold two positions depending on their individual qualifications. If for example the Chairperson is also qualified clinically or legally, then they may hold that position while serving as the Chairperson of the EC.

Alternate members of the EC may be appointed and will be subject to the same terms of reference as the Regular Members. Alternate Members may sit at a meeting and participate in all aspects of the meeting including decision making where a Regular Member cannot be present due to the requirement for a quorum.

The EC may establish a panel of Subject Experts (e.g., paediatricians for children's issues; cardiologists for heart-related matters) that can be called upon to give opinion on proposals submitted for consideration. The Subject Experts may provide the necessary expertise but would typically not vote on any proposal.

In some cases, the EC may invite independent consultants or special invitees, which could include representatives from patient groups (e.g., HIV/AIDS, Genetic Disorders, Cancer), to participate in deliberation on a particular issue or group of issues. Depending on the circumstances, these individuals may be given decision-making authority for a particular aspect of the deliberation.

Wherever possible, proposals for research projects should be reviewed by a separate scientific committee prior to being considered by the EC. However, it remains within the authority of the EC to raise questions concerning both the scientific merit and the ethical implications of any proposal. It is understood that the validity of the science and the integrity of the ethics are interconnected and therefore important to protect the welfare of participants and the quality of research outputs.

Standard 3: Resources for the Ethics Committee:

Administrative Support for Effective Operation of ECs:

Ethics Committees (ECs) require sufficient institutional support in order to operate autonomously and successfully. It is the responsibility of the authority that has established an EC to ensure that there are enough administrative, infrastructural and financial resources to allow the EC to perform its obligations effectively.

Support Staff for the EC:

These resources include providing qualified and experienced support staff to handle all documentation and correspondence related to the EC, including coordinating meetings and submissions and maintaining confidential records. In addition, the authority will need to provide the EC with a suitable office, secure storage facilities and required equipment, such as computers and communications tools, to provide for efficient administrative operations.

Meeting Venue and Communication Tools:

The authority will also need to provide the EC with access to a suitable meeting venue and reliable communication tools, such as telephones, e-mail and internet services to allow members of the EC to communicate efficiently and effectively.

Sustainable Funding:

Sufficient funding must be provided to the EC on a continuing basis to ensure that high-quality and efficient ethical review processes can continue to be conducted by the EC. This may include compensation to EC members for their time and expertise were deemed necessary. Adequate resources are essential for ensuring the credibility, accountability and effectiveness of the Ethics Committee.

Standard 4: Independence of the Ethics Committee:

To provide unbiased, fair, and trustworthy decision making, the Ethics Committee (EC) needs to be independent from any sponsor, investigator(s), or host organization involved in the research that it will be evaluating. Therefore, Institutional Policies need to clearly protect the EC from all external influences. In addition, no EC Member, including the Chairperson, can review any application where there is an apparent or potential Conflict of Interest involving themself or immediate family members.

Additionally, the EC must consist of at least one unaffiliated member with the sponsoring or conducting Institution. Investigators/Sponsors are allowed to attend committee meetings to answer questions, but they cannot participate during deliberations or final voting. The most senior institutional officials should not be members of the EC. Lastly, the members of the EC must be protected from any type of retaliation due to their ethical decisions.

Standard 5: Training of the Research Ethics Committee:

All REC members and staff need to take formal initial and ongoing education/training to be able to review health related research using human participants. The ICMR- National Institute for Research in Reproductive and Child Health emphasizes that all members will participate in a minimum of one training program every three years; however, they also encourage continuous professional development. Members who are new to the REC need to go through an orientation or induction training, and obtain copies of the institution's standard operating procedures (SOPs) as well as national ethical guidelines.

The training is based on the standards established by international and national organizations, which include the Council for International Organizations of Medical Sciences (CIOMS), the International Council for Harmonization of Technical Requirements for Pharmaceuticals for Human Use

(ICH) good clinical practice (GCP), the World Health Organization (WHO), and the Indian Council of Medical Research (ICMR). The training covers the key areas of: assessing risks versus benefits; evaluating vulnerabilities; understanding the process of obtaining informed consent; keeping current on changes in regulations; researching methods; and emerging issues such as research on stem cells, gene therapy, and public health emergencies. Secretariat support staff are provided additional training in the administrative functions of the EC, as well as the surveys that are used in the application process.

Committee members are expected to provide updated information they have learned from attending outside workshops to the rest of the committee. All travel expenses are paid for by the institution supporting the member, and all travel arrangements made for members are independent of any sponsors that may be involved in providing the training.

Terms of Reference and Selection Criteria for Ethics Committee Members:

Institutions need to make sure that all members of the Ethics Committee (including the Chairperson) are formally appointed by the Head of the Institution. The formal appointment letter must outline the Terms of Reference (TOR) for each member. A minimum requirement would include the roles/responsibilities of the member in relation to the EC, the duration of appointment and the conditions under which they can serve.

Membership of the EC typically has a duration of 2-3 years with the opportunity to extend in accordance with an institution's Standard Operating Procedures (SOPs). In order to facilitate both continuity and rotation of membership, a proportion of members will be rotated from time to time.

Institutions may provide reasonable compensation/honorarium for attendance at meetings of the EC, as a recognition of their time and expertise provided.

Each member of the EC must demonstrate their ability/ willingness to fulfill their responsibilities. Members must provide a recent signed CV, evidence of training in Human Research Protection, and if relevant, Good Clinical Practice (GCP) as part of the appointment process. Members that do not have the above training at the time of appointment must obtain the training within a set timeframe (usually within six months). Professional development is strongly encouraged throughout the term of the member.

Members of the EC must be familiar with the applicable ethical guidelines and regulatory requirements. Members must read, acknowledge and adhere to the EC's Conflict of Interest (COI) policy, declare any conflicts of interest when necessary, and sign confidentiality and COI agreements. There is a need for transparency and, therefore, members must agree to have their name, occupation and institutional affiliation publicly disclosed. Ultimately, members of the EC must protect participants, recognize the importance/value of conducting ethical research and uphold the principles of ethical research.

Appointments to the EC should be based on the individual's qualifications, experience, area of expertise and demonstrated interest in ethics oversight. Appointments are made in a personal capacity, and members must not act as a proxy for other individuals during EC meetings. Leadership positions such as Chairperson/Membership Secretary are additional areas of responsibility related to the individual's professional background. All criteria for appointments and function must be clearly outlined in an institution's SOPs to provide transparency and consistency.

Standard 6: Transparency, Accountability, and Quality of the Research Ethics Committee:

Transparency, accountability, and consistent quality are required for the operation of a Research Ethics Committee (REC). The parent institution will establish ways to ensure that REC policy and standard operating procedures are effectively carried out and that ethical standards in compliance with international and national guidelines are consistently applied. Internal evaluations of REC activity can occur on a periodic basis as part of a predetermined schedule using defined formats and may include independent, third-party evaluations.

The goal of these evaluations is to increase performance, enhance process, and increase public confidence in the REC, not to identify fault. Recommendations resulting from these evaluations must be seriously evaluated and acted upon.

The decisions of the REC, with the exception of confidential information, should be available to researchers and other stakeholders through established media outlets. In addition, research subjects and others must have avenues to report concerns or complaints about REC activities, with an independent entity making determinations regarding those complaints. Finally, open communication between researchers and REC members must be promoted.

Roles and Responsibilities of the EC:

the Ethics Committee (EC) is primarily accountable for ensuring that all participants in research have their rights, safety, dignity and welfare protected. Therefore, prior to approving any research proposal, the primary role of the Ethics Committee is to evaluate the scientific merit and ethical acceptability of proposals as well as the medical and social implications of conducting that research.

The Ethics Committee will assess whether participant informed consent procedures are adequate, understandable and voluntary; and provide additional safeguards for vulnerable groups (e.g., minors, elderly).

Furthermore, the Ethics Committee will evaluate the risk-benefit ratio of participating in the proposed research, ensure that the potential risks are minimized while justifying the potential benefits.

Additionally, the Ethics Committee will ensure that research studies are conducted according to universally recognized ethical principles and internationally accepted scientific standards in accordance with local cultural norms and community needs.

All members of the committee are required to disclose any conflicts of interest at each meeting and this disclosure must be properly documented.

The Ethics Committee will monitor and evaluate interim and final reports from researchers regarding study progress, protocol deviations, adverse events (AE/SAE) and final study reports to protect participants' welfare.

Where applicable, the Ethics Committee may recommend appropriate medical treatment or compensation to participants who experience injury as a result of participation in research.

The Ethics Committee also has the authority to conduct site visits ("monitoring") when necessary, maintain confidentiality of participant and study documents, discourage redundant ("me too") research and support ethics training within the institution.

Finally, the Ethics Committee promotes the harmonization of research practices and the secretariat provides administrative assistance in documenting, maintaining and ensuring compliance with confidentially agreements.

Submission and Review Procedures:

Researchers planning to conduct research should submit their proposals to the Ethics Committee (EC) Secretariat via the prescribed formats — electronically, or by printing them — along with all of the items listed in the EC's Standard Operating Procedures (SOPs), to ensure that the proposal is complete. The EC can maintain a current submission checklist for this purpose, which may need to be modified according to the study design, institutional policies, and regulatory requirements.

Documents Required for Ethical Review:

Typically, submissions are made up of: a covering letter addressed to the Member Secretary; information regarding what type of review is being requested; the completed application form; Informed Consent Documents, translated into English and/or the appropriate local language(s) along with proof of translation as needed; any necessary study aids (case report forms, questionnaires, etc.); materials used to recruit participants; participant instructions; Investigator's Brochure (for drug, biologic or device trials); Sponsor/Grantor information; Investigators Curriculum Vitae; Conflict of Interest Declarations; Recent GCP Certification for Clinical Trial Investigators; Evidence of any required Ethics Training; List of current projects for the Principal Investigator; Signed Investigator Undertaking; Regulatory and Administrative Approvals; Clearance for Stem Cell Research if applicable; Collaboration Agreements; Clinical Trial Agreement(s); Registration Information for the Trial; Participant Insurance and Indemnification Policies; Additional Clearances for Multicentre Trials; and the Complete Research Protocol.

Essential Components of the Protocol:

The study's protocol should provide the study title page with investigator signatures, a scientific summary of the study, an overview of the study including the justification and background, objectives, inclusion/exclusion criteria (including the rationale behind including vulnerable populations in this trial) and a description of how the study will be conducted with the number of participants to be included based on the rationale for that number, the overall study design, the specifics of the interventions used, the length of time the study will run, an evaluation of the potential risks and benefits of participating in the trial, the justification for using placebo in the study (if placebo is used), an explanation of how subjects will be informed of their rights as participants in the study (including whether there will be an audio or visual record of the subject being informed), a description of the statistical analysis plan for the study, the measures that will be taken to protect the confidentiality of the study participants, the procedures for managing injuries to study participants, the amount of compensation study participants will receive for their participation in the study, any other forms of care that will be provided to study participants, and how the data collected during the study will be stored and what policies will be followed regarding the publication of results from the study.

Categories of Review:

After submission, the Member Secretary or Secretariat screens proposals for completeness and classifies them according to risk into:

Exempt Review: Studies that have a risk level of minimal risk and will not contain any identifiers (either direct or indirect) can be exempted from a full Ethics Review by the Ethics Committee if participant anonymity and welfare are protected. Studies involving minimal risk are those studies in which there is a very small chance of adverse effects occurring; in other words, the probability of an adverse effect is so small it is essentially negligible, and the potential consequences of the adverse effects are so small they are negligible as well.

Further, studies in which participants cannot be identified by name or through data linkage may be exempt from full ethics review, even if the study involves participant interaction or some form of collection of private information.

Examples of studies that might meet this criterion include:

- Studies that rely solely on information that is available to the public and therefore do not require access to identifiable private information.
- Systematic reviews and meta-analyses that synthesize previously published data.

Since these types of studies do not involve contact with participants or access to identifiable private information, the ethical risk is believed to be extremely low.

Studies that involve observations of behaviour in public places, but only if the data collected is anonymous and if reporting of results would not likely cause harm to the people who were being observed, could also fit into this category. The two most important things to keep in mind regarding observational studies are that no personally identifiable information is collected and that the observation does not impinge upon the privacy rights of the people being observed.

Internal audits that are designed to evaluate and improve internal processes within an institution are generally viewed as having a low risk of harm to participants, especially if the audit does not collect identifiable personal data. Educational research that compares educational instruction methods, curricula or classroom management techniques may also be eligible, as long as no identifiable or sensitive information is collected.

Taste testing or consumer evaluation of food products, for example, qualify as low-risk as long as participation is voluntary and anonymous. Evaluations of public health programs conducted by a government agency, where the purpose of the evaluation is program improvement/monitoring and no individual identifiers are collected, may also be considered for exemption based on the lack of personal risk and the fact that the activity serves the public interest.

Expedited Review: In cases where the research presents minimal risk to participants, researchers have the option of submitting their proposal for an "expedited" review process instead of waiting for a full committee review meeting.

The expedited review process typically applies to studies that represent a low risk of potential injury or discomfort to participants. For example, studies that use non-identifiable biological materials, such as biological samples or tissue, collected from reputable sources like blood banks, tissue repositories, or leftover clinical samples with no linkable identifying information; studies that utilize non-identifiable clinical records, documents, or datasets, as long as confidentiality is adequately ensured; administrative corrections made to a study's original approval, such as correcting typographical errors, updating contact information, or replacing investigators who do not modify the scientific design of the study nor increase risk; revised submissions that were previously approved via either expedited or full review, as well as continued reviews of active studies that pose no additional risk to participants; minor protocol deviations that create no additional or substantial risks to participants; progress or annual reports, especially those studies that only analyze existing data and require no interaction with participants; and Serious Adverse Events (SAEs) or Unexpected Adverse Events that may be reviewed by a designated SAE subcommittee according to established policies and procedures.

Additionally, studies conducted at multiple sites may undergo a local Expedited Review in addition to the initial approval by the Central IRB, if all the necessary site-specific requirements have been met and approved by the Central IRB. The Expedited Review Process may also apply to studies initiated during emergencies or disasters, provided the research is performed ethically. Additionally, the expedited review process allows the institution to meet its obligations under federal regulations, as the expedited process was designed to provide an efficient means of reviewing research protocols while maintaining the high level of protection afforded to human subjects.

Full Committee Review: Institutional Review Board (IRB) Full Committee Reviews

The IRB will conduct full committee reviews for all new research studies that are defined as greater than minimal risk, involve vulnerable populations, include deception of participants, require a modification to the research protocol that could increase the risks of participants, require a major violation of any federal regulations, have serious safety concerns arising during the course of conducting the research, or if there is an urgent need to begin an emergency research project requiring thorough review.

Even though research projects that have been previously expedited must also be ratified by the full committee of the IRB, all proposed research studies which have been determined by the IRB to require full committee review will only be reviewed and voted upon by the full committee of the IRB at a duly convened full Institutional Review Board (IRB) meeting. Therefore, the IRB is expected to plan these meetings as part of a standard recurring schedule of meetings based on the IRB's Standard Operating Procedures (SOPs).

A meeting is considered a valid meeting only when a quorum is present, and this quorum must remain intact throughout the deliberations of the IRB and until a final determination is made. Should a member declare a conflict of interest (COI) prior to a meeting regarding a specific research project, it shall be documented in writing to the Chairperson of the IRB prior to the meeting commencing, and documented in the meeting minutes. In the event that a member declares a COI, the member will be asked to leave the meeting room during the discussion and voting process for the specific research project, but shall be noted in the minutes as having temporarily left the meeting room. Quorum must be re-established prior to continuing discussions on the project.

Attendance records are valuable for maintaining transparency and accountability of the decision-making process. Meeting minutes should document attendance of the members attending the meeting, as well as documentation of any members who enter or leave the meeting mid-stream. Research proposals should be reviewed in sequence as presented in the approved meeting agenda. A reasonable number of research projects should be included in the meeting agenda to allow adequate time for a meaningful discussion of each research project submission. If the IRB workload becomes excessive, more frequent meetings can be scheduled, or additional IRBs can be established within the institution, contingent upon the needs of the institution. Sufficient time must be allowed for a meaningful discussion of each research project submission on the agenda.

Prior to commencing the meeting, the minutes from the preceding meeting should be reviewed and validated by the committee. In addition, research projects that were classified as exempt or reviewed using expedited procedures since the last meeting must be formally ratified by the full committee of the IRB.

Invitations may be extended to researchers to present their research proposals and/or to clarify questions raised about their submitted research protocol; however, researchers are not permitted to attend the committee's deliberations and/or make the final decisions. It is the responsibility of the primary reviewer(s) and secondary reviewer(s) assigned to a research project to summarize the researcher's proposal and to present their assessment(s) of the research project as outlined in the IRB's SOPs.

If the IRB has requested input from an independent consultant regarding a particular research project, the comments of the independent consultant may be presented by the Member Secretary of the IRB, or the consultant may be invited to provide further clarification regarding his/her comments. Subject matter experts, as well as representatives of the study population, may be invited to provide insights and/or perspectives that relate to the research project being reviewed. Regardless, such individuals are not permitted to vote nor influence the final decision of the committee. Their contributions, when made, should be documented in the meeting minutes.

When deemed necessary, the IRB may utilize electronic communication technologies, such as video conferencing, to obtain the input of subject matter experts. All committee members in attendance during the deliberations of the committee, including the Chairperson and Member Secretary, are entitled to offer their opinions and to vote.

The IRB shall arrive at a final determination regarding each research project submission through consensus or by a majority vote as outlined in the IRB's SOPs. The outcome of the review of each research project submission must be clearly documented in the meeting minutes, and any dissenting opinions and/or rationale for those dissenting opinions must also be documented in the meeting minutes.

Researchers cannot self-assign the review category; the EC determines this on a case-by-case basis. Expedited decisions must be confirmed at the subsequent full meeting.

Standard 7: Ethical Basis for Decision-Making and Ethical Issues in Protocol Review:

Ethics committee decisions must always be made by reference to a well-defined set of ethical principles, based upon internationally accepted guidelines, nationally mandated rules and human rights. The ethics committee must also make it clear through its framework, documentation, and consistent application how those principles will be used to inform all of its decision-making. Although when an ethics committee is responsible for reviewing matters on behalf of others, it may delegate some responsibility to others to conduct reviews, it is still accountable for ensuring that the same high ethical standard is utilised. Any deviation from the previously established interpretation of an ethical principle must have a valid explanation and be documented, to provide a basis for maintaining the consistency and integrity of decision-making.

Social and Scientific Value of Research:

Public health must be a significant focus of research in order for it to have social relevance and benefits to public health. Therefore, a study with no inherent value cannot ethically be conducted. Scientific validity also needs to be demonstrated; studies with methodological flaws expose participants to avoidable risks. Consequently, the EC must evaluate whether there are sufficient study design, sample size, feasibility and investigators' ability to produce valid results.

Risk–Benefit Assessment:

A thorough evaluation of potential risks and anticipated benefits is central to ethical review. Risks—physical, psychological, social, or economic—must be minimized and proportionate to expected benefits. Plans for safety monitoring, management of adverse events, and compensation for research-related injury must be clearly described.

Fair Participant Selection and Protection of Vulnerable Groups:

Participant recruitment should be equitable and based on scientific objectives, not convenience or vulnerability. Special safeguards are required when including populations with limited autonomy. Participation must always be voluntary, with the right to withdraw without penalty.

Informed Consent Process:

The EC must carefully review how consent will be obtained, ensuring that information is clear, culturally appropriate, and comprehensive. Consent must reflect genuine understanding and voluntariness. Waivers or alterations of consent require strong ethical justification.

Privacy, Confidentiality, and Data Protection:

Adequate measures must be in place to protect personal information and prevent misuse or disclosure of sensitive data. Secure data storage and confidentiality safeguards are essential.

Financial Considerations and Undue Influence:

Payments or reimbursements should compensate for time and expenses without exerting undue influence on participation.

Community Considerations and Cultural Sensitivity:

Research should respect cultural values and avoid stigmatizing communities. Engagement strategies should promote transparency and social responsibility.

Conflict of Interest Management:

Investigators and EC members must disclose potential conflicts of interest. Appropriate steps should be taken to prevent bias in decision-making.

Through adherence to these ethical foundations, the EC ensures that research review remains rigorous, fair, and protective of participant rights while promoting scientifically sound and socially valuable research.

Deliberation and Decision-Making Process:

Investigators are sometimes asked to discuss their proposals during ethics committee (EC) meeting review sessions; however, to maintain objectivity, the investigator must leave prior to the voting portion of the review session. Primary and secondary reviewers from designated positions will describe the proposed research, as well as evaluate it according to the established standard operating procedures (SOPs).

Independent consultant(s)/subject matter experts may be used if specialized knowledge is required. In addition, representatives of the study population can be contacted to provide relevant information about the study population. While these individuals' comments are important and should be documented, they will have no role in decision making.

Ethics Committee decisions are made by all committee members who are present at the time of decision making (i.e., the chairperson and member secretary); therefore, all members will have an opportunity to comment/vote regarding the decision (e.g., consensus or majority vote). All dissenting comments along with rationale must be documented. The EC may:

Approve a submission (with or without recommendations),

Grant conditional approval (with minor revisions),

Require major changes and resubmit for full review, or

Reject/terminate approval (with clear justification).

In some cases, approval for a study will be given for the duration of the study; however, in other cases, the study may need to undergo annual/periodic reviews depending upon the type of study and the level of risk associated with the study. Prior to continuing the study, all annual reports must be reviewed.

Monitoring of Approved Research and Appeals:

A number of factors can influence how often a monitoring schedule is required; the frequency will depend on the level of risk involved, which could be at intervals such as annually, semi-annually, or quarterly. Approval to continue is dependent upon satisfactory progress; however, should new data result in a revision to the benefit/risk assessment by the EC, they have the ability to either reconsider their previous approval of the research, or withdraw that approval entirely.

The Member Secretary and the Secretariat record the detail of all discussions in formal minutes, and circulate them to other members for comment prior to the minutes being approved by the Chairperson, or their designated authority. Once decisions are made and recommendations are provided to the researcher, formal notification of the decision(s) and recommendation(s), including the rationale for same, are provided to the investigator. A reasonable amount of time is allowed for researchers to respond to any concerns or questions raised by the EC, and/or to provide additional clarification to the EC. Should there still be disagreement(s), the investigator may appeal to the institutional head (the Appellate Authority); the institutional head, in addition to making a determination on the appeal, also has the option to reconstitute the EC or dissolve it if necessary.

Review of Multicentric Research:

Multicentre trials, conducted in several locations using the same protocol, are required to have ethical clearance from all participating centres so that local cultural, social, and regulatory needs can be addressed. Coordination and communication among the various ethics committees (ECs) at different locations is encouraged in order to avoid duplicate reviews and improve the effectiveness of coordinating approvals. Reasons for denial of approval at any one centre should be provided to the other centres to allow for discussion and potential modifications to the trial protocol and/or informed consent document to accommodate local requirements. Modifications may include changes to the informed consent document as well as the introduction of additional safety measures at specific centres.

For low-risk multicentre trials, it is possible for participating ECs to designate a primary EC whose decisions will be accepted by the other ECs involved. However, representatives from each EC involved in the trial may also attend meetings of the designated primary EC to discuss and resolve concerns. In addition, each individual EC retains the authority to establish site-specific safeguards, to monitor compliance with those safeguards, and to take action if necessary.

While the use of a common review process may apply to trials conducted solely in India, an additional level of review is required when conducting trials internationally (i.e., outside of India). Therefore, sponsors must obtain local ethical approval prior to initiating any international multicentre trial and they must also inform the other participating ECs of any site-specific changes that are made during the course of the trial. Agreement on publication plans, and the format of a consolidated final report must be reached prior to the initiation of the study. Publication of site level data must be accompanied by the appropriate permissions.

Continuing Review of Ongoing Research:

All studies must go through a periodic evaluation process - at least once a year or more often if needed - based on how risky they are, as stated in the SOPs. The EC will evaluate the progress reports, SAEs, any protocol deviations, any incidents of non-compliance and any new safety concerns related to the study. For all clinical trials, compliance with any applicable SAE reporting requirements is mandatory. The policies of the institution will direct academic or unregulated studies.

The EC must also provide appropriate medical care for any study related injuries and pay for any expenses the participant incurred because of their injury. If it is required by law or by the EC, compensation must be paid when warranted. In cases of serious protocol violations the EC has the right to stop the study and submit chronic non-compliance to institutional and/or government entities. Monitoring reports from the sponsor and Data Safety Monitoring Boards (DSMBs) will also be evaluated.

Site Monitoring:

Monitoring of ethics committee-approved research sites is necessary to ensure that studies are conducted in accordance with established protocols and protect participants from harm. The ethics committee's standard operating procedure (SOP) will outline the parameters for conducting such monitoring activities. These monitoring activities can include either routine monitoring or "for cause" monitoring due to some concern(s) identified during the review process. More frequent monitoring of those studies considered to involve greater risks, vulnerable populations, and/or other safety concerns may be required to assure compliance with approved study protocols, continue to protect the rights and welfare of participants, and ensure public trust.

For-Cause Monitoring:

When "for-cause" monitoring begins due to issues related to the way a study was conducted, that process can occur if the research team has demonstrated a pattern of violating or deviating from the protocol; if a location or an investigator are conducting too many studies; if the rate of reporting of SAEs is too high; if recruitment appears to be occurring rapidly enough; if adverse media attention arises; or if the research team receives negative feedback from any legitimate source. Any type of non-adherence to directives issued by the EC, any allegations or evidence of research misconduct by investigators, and participant complaint(s) further justify "for-cause" monitoring. The EC also maintains the right to monitor for any reason it determines necessary to protect participants' rights, safety and welfare.

Standard 9: Written Policies and Procedures:

A Research Ethics Committee (REC) has to follow well-defined policy and standard operating procedures (SOP) that outline the structure, authority, and operation of the REC. These written policies will serve as a basis for a fair, equitable, and accountable ethics review process; they include but are not limited to:

- Composition of the REC
- Governance
- Review Processes
- Decision Making Processes
- Communication Processes
- Continuing Oversight
- Documentation Practices
- Training Requirements
- Quality Assurance Processes
- Coordination with Other RECs

Appropriate institutional policies must be established by the host institution to guide the operation of the REC. The REC formally accepts and adopts rules of procedure, and collaborates with the Secretariat or Support Staff to develop detailed written SOPs. These policies and procedures should be provided to each member of the REC and be available to the public for transparency purposes. The host institution is responsible for providing an adequately trained Secretariat that has the knowledge and expertise necessary to facilitate the ethics review activities, recordkeeping, and administrative coordination of the REC. Policies and Procedures should be reviewed and revised at least annually, based upon evaluations of performance and changing regulatory or ethical standards.

Membership of the Committee:

Clearly defined policies on member appointments need to include information about the basis for their appointment (i.e., the authority), the criteria they will use for evaluation of candidates for membership, and the conditions under which a candidate will be appointed. Ideally, the length of service or "term" should be set as a fixed number and staggered so that some members are appointed at the same time each year, ensuring there is always continuity in the group, and that at least a few new faces are introduced regularly. Fixed terms can foster more overall growth of expertise in research ethics throughout the institution, as well as introduce different viewpoints into the committee's decision-making process.

Committee Governance:

Written procedure will have to include the organizational chart for the REC and will have to clearly define what the Chairperson and Vice-Chairperson are responsible for in terms of their duties. It is preferable that the Chairperson is neutral so as to provide a forum for constructive dialogue, provide an opportunity to bring forth different perspectives, and lead the group towards a common point of view. The position of Chairperson should not be given to someone who has direct supervision of some or all of the committee members. This would help prevent any potential conflict of interest with regards to the ability of the committee to make independent decisions.

Use of Independent Consultants:

In order to protect its independence, an REC's policies must define circumstances in which the REC can seek outside expertise. When a researcher is conducting studies that require special knowledge (e.g., those involving unusual or untested procedures), special populations (e.g., children, prisoners) or ethics issues of some complexity, it may be appropriate to invite outside advisors who are knowledgeable about these issues. These advisors provide information to the REC as needed and should not take over the decision making function of the REC; rather they should assist the REC to make informed decisions based on the best available data.

Submission Requirements, Review Procedures, and Decision-Making:

Beginning with standard operating procedures (SOPs) for routine operations, SOPs must include processes for submitting research proposals. This includes which forms should be submitted, which additional documentation should accompany those forms, which process to follow when reviewing the proposed research in a sequential manner, how to ensure coordination among committee members, the method for notifying attendees of upcoming meetings, and the process by which materials will be distributed to the attendees; the eligibility requirements to participate as a non-committee member (invited member); and the approval of meeting minutes. In addition to these details, it is essential that the decision-making and deliberation processes be clearly outlined in the SOPs, as well as a definition of what constitutes a quorum, so that a legitimate review/decision may take place.

Communication of Decisions:

Policies must establish how and within what timeframe decisions are communicated to applicants. Clear timelines between final determination and formal notification ensure predictability and accountability in the review process.

Follow-Up Review and Monitoring:

SOPs should outline mechanisms for ongoing oversight of approved research, beginning from the date of approval and continuing until study completion or termination. This includes procedures for reviewing progress reports, safety updates, and compliance with approved protocols.

Record Keeping and Archiving:

Active and closed study files are to be kept separate and labelled appropriately in designated storage areas. Study records may be stored in either paper or electronic format if sufficient safeguards, such as secured cabinets, passwords, and encryption, are used to protect them. Study related records are to be stored for at least three years after completion of the study or until the end of the study. However, in the case of regulated clinical studies, all study related records are to be stored for a minimum of five years and up to the time required by law or by the sponsor agreement. The EC SOPs shall detail how the study records will be stored and how they can be retrieved. In addition, the study records are to be made available for review by the regulatory representative. When possible, electronic systems for storing records may be utilized to provide an efficient and secure method of record keeping.

Documents to be Maintained by the EC:

Administrative files are required to contain information that defines the constitution and membership of the EC as well as appointment letters, updated and signed CV's, Confidentiality Agreements, Declarations of Interest in Conflict of Interest, Training Records, and Financial Documents.

Additionally, registration/accreditation certificates, national/international guidelines/guidance documents, Regulatory Correspondence, Meeting Agenda's & Minutes, Official Correspondence, and Standard Operating Procedures (SOPs) will need to be maintained.

Proposal files are to include both physical and electronic versions of the submitted Research Proposal(s), as well as all supporting documentation. Files must also include Decision Letters, Approved Amendments, Regulatory Permissions, Reports of Adverse Events, Deviations from Protocol, Progress Reports, Continuing Review Documents, Site Monitoring Reports, and All Correspondence between the EC and Investigators.

Finally, Documentation related to Premature Study Termination; Reasons for termination, Final Study Report, and Any Resulting Publications will also be part of the archive.

Administration and Management:

All institutions need to create an independent office for the EC to have enough physical room, equipment and personnel to be able to employ a full-time administrative team. All institutions will also need to set aside suitable rooms and equipment that is appropriate for storing sensitive records securely, and to meet with all interested parties. Each institution will be responsible for setting aside a suitable budget to allow the EC to function effectively. The institution can charge a reasonable document review fee as required by its internal policies to cover its costs in providing support services for the EC.

Registration and Accreditation of ECs:

Ethics Committees are required to develop an infrastructure for ensuring that ethical review is conducted at the highest level possible; maintaining the quality and integrity of the ethical review process; and complying with all pertinent national and international laws, regulations, standards and guidelines. A registration with the relevant National Regulatory Authority is a requirement under current law. In addition, it is highly recommended that ECs seek voluntary recognition/ accreditation by a reputable National or International Body as this will add strength to their Quality Assurance Mechanisms. The Recognition/Accreditation shall be subject to renewal on a periodic basis to ensure that the EC continues to adhere to Best Practices for Protecting the Dignity, Rights, Safety and Well Being of Research Participants.

Standard 10: Researchers' Responsibilities:

Research may be conducted by only those that have the appropriate education and qualifications for a particular project, such as scientific, clinical or other related professions. These professionals are also expected to have knowledge of the ethical guidelines and regulations associated with the proposed research and provide all necessary information to the Research

Ethics Committee (REC) for review. This includes all information pertaining to the research proposal (protocol) and any possible conflict of interests that may exist. Upon receiving approval from the REC, these professionals will then conduct the research according to the terms and requirements outlined by the REC.

Submitting an Application for Ethical Review:

A researcher will need to submit an ethics review application to determine if there are ethical issues in his/her proposed study. The researcher must assume primary responsibility for the scientific integrity and the ethical conduct of this research. In some jurisdictions, the study sponsor is responsible for submitting the application to the Research Ethics Committee (REC) and in others, the applicant is required to submit the application as part of the requirements for conducting research. When the researcher is a student, he/she must submit the application with a qualified faculty advisor that provides academic and professional supervision. The advisor has shared responsibility for the study and is expected to sign off on or formally support the submission of the application. The researcher must provide all documentation that is needed to complete an ethical review of their study. This includes but is not limited to, study protocol, participant information document, consent forms, and disclosure of any potential financial or personal conflict of interest.

Conduct of Research:

Researchers have an obligation to carry out the study according to the exact protocol approved by the REC. Researchers can only make changes to the approved study protocol with prior approval from the REC, unless the researcher has to immediately make some changes to protect the well-being of the participants. If a researcher has to immediately modify the protocol to protect the participants' well-being, then the researcher must inform the REC of this action as soon as possible. The researcher must provide the REC with a detailed explanation of why they had to deviate from the approved protocol. Researchers must also inform the REC if there is any material change at the research site that could potentially endanger the participants' safety, change the risk/benefit ratio of participating in the study, or impact the participants' access to the services/care that were promised during the recruitment process.

Safety Reporting:

All serious and unexpected adverse event(s) related to the trial and all other unforeseen issues of risk to subjects or third parties must be notified immediately to the REC and the appropriate regulatory authority as per current guidelines and law. The researcher is to take immediate action on any recommendations/ remedial actions that may be identified by the REC based on their notification of these adverse event(s)/ unforeseen issue(s).

Ongoing Reporting and Follow-Up:

Researchers are required to submit to the REC periodic written updates on the research's progress and its status; these updates should occur at least once per year, but may need to happen more often at the request of the REC. When the researcher has completed their study, either temporarily or permanently suspended it, or terminated it, the researcher is also required to notify the REC of the reason for such an action. When a researcher or sponsor initiates an early suspension or termination of the study, the REC will be notified of the reasons for the termination, provided with a summary of the findings collected thus far, and notified of how the results will be communicated to participants, and how they will be followed up after the conclusion of the study. If the REC decides to withdraw approval for the research or suspend approval of the research, the researcher is required to communicate this decision to the host institution, to the sponsor, and to other entities that have a vested interest in the outcome of the study.

Information to Research Participants:

Researchers have a continuing obligation to inform participants (and, as appropriate, participants' communities) of major developments in the research. Communication should be timely and in non-technical terms. Participants should be informed of any discontinuance of the study, of any new information that may have altered potential risk and benefit, at the conclusion of the project, and at such time as findings are made available.

References:

1. World Health Organization. (2000). *Operational guidelines for ethics committees that review biomedical research.* https://www.who.int/tdr/publications/documents/ethics.pdf

2. International Conference on Harmonisation of Technical Requirements for Registration of Pharmaceuticals for Human Use. (1996). *Guideline for good clinical practice (ICH-GCP).* https://www.ich.org/LOB/media/MEDIA482.pdf

3. Indian Council of Medical Research. (2018). *National ethical guidelines for biomedical and health research involving*

human participants. https://ethics.ncdirindia.org/asset/pdf/Handbook_on_ICMR_Ethical_Guidelines.pdf

4. Government of India. (2006). *Drugs and Cosmetics Act, 1940 and Rules, 1945 (Schedule Y amendment, December 31, 2006)*. https://cdsco.gov.in/opencms/export/sites/CDSCO_WEB/Pdfdocuments/acts_rules/2016DrugsandCosmeticsAct1940Rules1945.pdf

Declaration of Originality and Conflict of Interest:

I hereby declare that this content is original and has been prepared based on the following primary sources:

World Health Organization. (2000). *Operational guidelines for ethics committees that review biomedical research.*

Indian Council of Medical Research. (2018). *National ethical guidelines for biomedical and health research involving human participants.*

The work has not been published previously and is not under consideration elsewhere. I declare that there are no financial or personal conflicts of interest that could have influenced this work.

Chapter 8

Good Clinical Practice and Clinical Trial

Dr Emmanuel Bhaskar
Professor, Department of Medicine
Sri Ramachandra Medical College, Porur, Chennai
drebhaskar@sriramachandra.edu.in

Abstract:

This chapter provides an overview of clinical trials, their phases, and the principles of Good Clinical Practice (GCP). It outlines the design, conduct, and ethical safeguards of clinical trials, along with the roles and responsibilities of investigators, sponsors, ethics committees, and regulatory authorities. Emphasis is placed on participant safety, informed consent, scientific validity, and data integrity. The chapter highlights that adherence to GCP ensures ethical conduct, reliability of results, and protection of human subjects in clinical research.

Keywords:

Clinical Trials; Good Clinical Practice; GCP; Study Phases; Ethics; Informed Consent; Investigator; Sponsor; Ethics Committee; Regulatory Authority

Objectives:

- Understand the concept and phases of clinical trials
- Describe roles of stakeholders in clinical research
- Explain principles of Good Clinical Practice
- Apply ethical and scientific standards in clinical trials

Definition of Clinical Trials and Phases of Clinical Trials:

What is a Clinical Trial?

A clinical trial is a scientifically designed study conducted in human participants to evaluate the safety, efficacy, and optimal use of a medical intervention. The intervention is mostly a drug or vaccine, but it can be a medical device, a surgical procedure or even a diagnostic test or a lifestyle modification.

This is different from usual clinical care in which the goal of the clinician is to treat an individual patient with a well-established treatment. In clinical trial, the intervention used has to be monitored since it is yet to be proven to be effective and its safety is not fully known.

A clinical trial generally has an outline with the following in mind. It is prepared by the person who initiates the study. Most drug studies are initiated by the drug company who is called the sponsor of the study. But the clinical trial can also be initiated by an individual academic researcher or a research institute. Even in sponsor study the actual study is carried out by an independent clinician who is given financial assistance by the company but given the freedom to decide without interference from the company.

Let us now see a brief overview of the components of a clinical trial document.

1. Study objectives: This lays down the main objective of the intervention which is called the primary objective. Some studies have secondary objectives which are not the main outcome assessed, but are looked to plan follow-up studies.

2. Eligibility criteria: This mentions details of patients who are included (example: age > 18 years, diabetic, etc) or excluded (age > 70 years, presence of chronic kidney disease, etc)

3. Intervention details: This explains the details of what is tested for its benefits as well as safety. It can be a drug or any other we have seen in the definition of a clinical trial. All details of the intervention need to be mentioned(drug preparation, dose, route of administration, monitoring, etc). Sometimes, a placebo is given in the comparative group. In that case, details of the placebo material should be disclosed (colour, form, if similar in looks to study drug)

4. Outcome measures: This is the goal of the study. Like improvement in blood sugar with a new drug compared to an existing drug.

5. Statistical plan: Calculation of sample size before the start of the study is essential to plan the duration of the study, number of centres to be included, etc. The sample size is calculated based on previous data from observational studies with the intervention, or on presumptive rates from pre-clinical use.

6. Ethical safeguards: This caries information on how the study participants will be protected from harm. It has the

patient information sheet which explains to the participant or to their parents in case of children or to their legal guardians in case of sick or mentally challenged patients. This forms the basis of the informed consent signed by the participant or their guardian. It will be in the local language. Others included along with the document is the travel compensation which will be given, and how the participant will be taken care if any side effect of the intervention is observed.

What are the Phases of Clinical Trials?

Before a new drug, device or vaccine is used for treatment in regular clinical practice, it undergoes testing in the laboratory, followed by studies in animals and then in a small number of patients. But clinical trials are essential to find if that intervention is safe and whether it actually works. If it works then is any side effects, what is the safe dose and more such questions.

During the COVID-19 pandemic, vaccines such as using mRNA technology was ready within 6 months of the pandemic. But it took over a year to confirm whether it was safe for human use. This duration in-fact very short. Generally, it takes 4 to 5 years of clinical trials before an intervention is approved for use in regular practice.

So there are phases to be followed before the drug is approved and modifications are made after every phase based on the findings.

Phases of Clinical Trials

Typically there are 4 phases (Phase I to IV). Each phase has a clear objective and also a defined study population

Phase I: Is the safety and dose finding phase. The objective is to assess the tolerability and safety of a particular dose and arrive at the desirable dose. A small number of participants are included. In clinical trials on cancer, they are tested in about 20 to 100 patients. This phase answers on the dose of the drug , how body metabolises it and if there are any immediate side effects of the new drug.

Example: A new anti-diabetic drug is tested in 20 human volunteers to see how the medicine is absorbed and if causes low blood sugar levels more than what is expected from it.

Phase II: Is the preliminary efficacy and safety study. This evaluated the effectiveness and gathers more information on the safety. A higher number of participants are enrolled (n=100 to 300). Here the focus will be on questions like does the drug work? These trials are often randomized controlled trial which ensure that the study group and the comparative group are equally balanced. Each eligible patient included in the study have equal change of entering the study or comparative group. The choice of group is made by tossing a coin or by opening an envelope that has the group assignment details. Now the enrolment is computer-generated. The duration is longer than the Phase I trial. This phase gives more clarity on the range of dose, side effects which are seen after a delay and also gives the preliminary evidence of benefit.

Example: The anti-diabetic drug is now tested in 200 patients with mild Type 2 diabetes to see whether it lowers HbA1c levels compared to a placebo or an existing drug.

If the findings of the Phase II study is favourable and the drug is safe to be used in a larger group, the drug proceeds to Phase III. However, the group which is planning to do the Phase

III need to get the permission of the regulatory bodies before proceeding further. In India , Central Drugs Standard Control Organization (CDSCO) is the regulatory agency which oversees all clinical trials.

Phase III: This phase includes Confirmatory Trials where the efficiency of the drug is confirmed and rates of adverse events in a larger population is studied. These are also randomized control trials and are done on a larger population (1000 to 3000) often involving multiple centres across the world. The duration is usually more than 3 years. The results of this phase forms the basis of regulatory approval for use in humans.

Example: The anti-diabetic drug is now used in patients with higher blood sugar at baseline and compared with metformin or other diabetic drug in 2,500 patients across multiple countries to evaluate how much does the long term sugar control occurs, long tern safety and if any other organ benefits or harm occur.

If Phase III results show benefit and acceptable safety, regulatory authorities may approve the drug. But a surveillance study should be initiated.

Phase IV: This phase is called Post-Marketing Surveillance since the focus is on long-term safety and to identify rare adverse events. The population will be from real-world practice settings, diverse patient groups where drug interactions will be known

Example: During the study if there is a small percentage of pancreatitis then the drug may not be withdrawn , but used with caution in a group of patients who may develop the complication.

Many drugs have been withdrawn during Phase IV due to unexpected serious adverse effects.

Recognize Roles and Responsibilities of Investigators, Sponsors, Institutional Ethics Committees and Regulatory Bodies:

When we speak about a clinical trial, many students imagine that it is only about the doctor and the patient. But in real world , a clinical trial is a coordinated effort involving multiple stakeholders. Each person or body has clearly defined roles. If one fails, the safety of participants and the scientific validity of the study may be compromised.

Let us now understand clearly who these stakeholders are and what exactly they are responsible for.

1. The Investigator:

The Investigator is the person who actually conducts the clinical trial at the study site. Usually, this is a qualified medical practitioner. In many multicentric trials, there is a Principal Investigator (PI) at each site and sometimes a Co-Investigator or Sub-Investigator to assist.

Who appoints the investigator?

In sponsor-initiated studies, the sponsor selects investigators based on clinical expertise and research experience since all clinicians may not have the ability to conduct a research. Another factor would be the availability of the necessary infrastructure like storage of the experimental drug, research assistants who assist the investigator on patient appointment , office staff to maintain patient records, etc. The final, but a very important one is patient availability. Patients with common illness like diabetes mellitus is easy to get, but conditions like pancreatic cancers are often available only in centres which handle large volume of such cases.

But after the sponsor identifies the investigator and once the study begins, the investigator functions independently in the interest of patient safety.

Responsibilities of the Investigator will include

1. Protecting the Rights, Safety and Well-being of Participants: This is the most important responsibility. The investigator must ensure that the participant understands the study, including the benefits and risks before getting the informed consent. More than getting the signature, the investigator should be convinced that the participant understood the study and have cleared all their doubts before getting enrolled in the study. If patient feels uncomfortable in continuing in the study and wishes to withdraw, the investigator should not hesitate to permit the patient to withdraw from the study.

2. Reporting of serious adverse events: Any adverse events which occur to the patient after getting enrolled in the study should be assessed by the investigator and treated as per best medical practice. The initial cost of the treatment should be borne by the sponsor till the causal association of the adverse event to the drug is excluded. If the adverse event is serious like requiring hospitalization , it should be reported to the sponsor and the institutional ethics committee which approved the study. It should be reported within 24 hours of the occurrence of the serious adverse effect. Less serious adverse effects are recorded in the patient case forms and discussed later. If the serious adverse effect has occurred as a result of the study drug, then the entire treatment expense is borne by the sponsor and a

compensation as recommended by the ethics committee is given to the participant.

3. Conducting the Study as per Protocol: A clinical trial is conducted according to a predefined protocol. The investigator:

    - Must follow the inclusion and exclusion criteria strictly.
    - Ensure that the drug is administered in the appropriate dose.
    - Maintain proper documentation of all trial related medical and patient related facts in the patient medical records and takes appropriate action as and when required.

4. Avoid protocol deviations unless necessary for safety. For example, if the protocol says only patients aged 18–65 can be included, enrolling a patient without proof of date of birth is a protocol violation. If a patient is supposed to review at 1 week after starting the test drug and he reviews after 2 weeks, then it is a protocol deviation. All deviations in protocol should be reported to the sponsor and the ethics committee.

5. Ensuring Proper Informed Consent. Informed consent is not just a signature on paper. The investigator must explain the study in simple language, discuss risks and benefits, allow time for questions by the patient or their guardian. Provide the patient information sheet in the local language. In India, consent must be documented properly, and in some studies audiovisual recording may be required.

6. Maintaining Study Records: The investigator must maintain, Case record forms (CRFs), adverse events record, drug

accountability records which mentioned details of used and unused drugs, and travel compensation payment records. A good documentation ensures transparency and audit readiness.

7. Communication with Sponsor and Ethics Committee: The investigator must report adverse events as appropriate for the seriousness of the event. Submit periodic progress reports to sponsor and ethics committee on the trial status. Seek approval for protocol amendments from ethics committee. Inform about study completion to ethics committee.

2. The Sponsor:

Responsibilities of the Sponsor

The Sponsor is the individual, company, institution, or organization that initiates, manages, and finances the clinical trial. In most drug trials, the sponsor is a pharmaceutical company. However, academic institutions, government agencies, or independent researchers may also act as sponsors.

Let us now understand what the sponsor is responsible for.

1. Designing and monitoring the Study: The sponsor develops: The study protocol , which describes the purpose of the study and the methods. Investigator brochure, which elaborates on the details of the study drug or device which is about to be used in the study. Statistical analysis plan which describes the total number of participants to be enrolled and details of statistical test planned after the data collection

is completed. Monitoring plan of the entire study with respect to accuracy of data collection, speed of recruitment of population, safety of the participants and action to be taken when adverse events occur. Most sponsors form a Safety and Monitoring board which supervise the entire process of the study.

2. Regulatory Approval: Before starting the trial, the sponsor must obtain approval from regulatory authorities (e.g., CDSCO in India). Following the government regulatory Ethics committee approvals at each site is required. Only after both these approvals , the clinical trial can be started.

3. Selecting Qualified Investigators: As already discussed the sponsor must ensure that the Investigators are qualified, sites have adequate infrastructure and necessary equipment is available.

4. Providing Investigational Product: The sponsor is responsible for manufacturing the investigational drug. Ensuring quality and stability. Labelling properly. Supplying it to study sites. They must maintain accountability of study drug.

5. Safety Reporting The sponsor must collect safety data from all sites. Analyse adverse events. Report serious unexpected adverse reactions to regulatory authorities.

6. Compensation and Insurance

In India, the sponsor must provide compensation for trial-related injury and arrange insurance coverage. Follow compensation rules as per regulatory guidelines. This is a critical ethical responsibility.

3. Institutional Ethics Committee (IEC):

The Institutional Ethics Committee (IEC) is an independent body that safeguards the rights and welfare of participants. No clinical trial can begin without IEC approval.

Composition of IEC:

An IEC typically includes:

- Chairperson (clinician or basic scientist, external member)
- Clinician (internal member, who can also act as member secretary)
- Basic scientist (internal members, preferably a pharmacologist, who can also be a member secretary)
- Legal expert (external member)
- Social scientist/ worker(external member)
- Lay person (external member)

This diverse composition ensures balanced decision-making.

Responsibilities of IEC:

aEthical Review of Protocol: The IEC evaluates scientific validity of the study and assesses the Risk-benefit ratio , Inclusion of vulnerable populations , Adequacy of informed consent. If risk outweighs benefit, approval may be denied.

i. Review of Informed Consent Documents : IEC checks Language clarity , Local language translation, Compensation details, Voluntary participation statement and if the participant's autonomy is respected.

ii. Monitoring Ongoing Studies IEC does not give approval and stop with it. It must review periodic progress reports. Review serious adverse events. Review protocol deviations. Conduct continuing review (usually annually).

iii. Protection of Vulnerable Populations Special care is required for Children , Pregnant women Mentally challenged individuals, Economically disadvantaged groups, and frail elderly. IEC ensures they are not exploited.

4. Regulatory Bodies:

Regulatory bodies are government authorities that oversee clinical trials at a national level. In India, the regulatory authority is the Central Drugs Standard Control Organization (CDSCO) under the Drug Controller General of India (DCGI).

Other examples: US: FDA (Food and Drug Administration) Europe: EMA (European Medicines Agency)

Responsibilities of Regulatory Bodies:

1. Granting Permission to Conduct Trials Before Phase II and Phase III trials especially, regulatory approval is mandatory.

   They review: Preclinical data, Phase I data , Manufacturing quality, Safety information .

2. Oversight and Inspection : Regulators conduct site inspections, Audit of documentation, Review of safety reports. If violations occur, they can suspend the trial , Cancel approval and Impose penalties

3. Approving Marketing Authorization: After successful Phase III trials, regulatory bodies decide whether the drug can be marketed.

4. Post-Marketing Surveillance: Oversight even after approval, regulators monitor pharmacovigilance data. Review adverse drug reactions. Withdraw drugs if needed. Many drugs worldwide have been withdrawn after post-marketing reports revealed rare but serious adverse effects.

How All Stakeholders Work Together:

Let us understand this with a simple example. Suppose a new anti-hypertensive drug is being tested. The Sponsor designs and funds the study. The Regulatory Authority approves it to begin. The IEC evaluates ethical aspects. The Investigator recruits patients and conducts the trial. If a patient develops liver injury, the investigator treats the patient and reports it. Sponsor analyses safety data. IEC reviews whether the trial should continue. The regulatory body may intervene if the risk is high. This system ensures multiple layers of protection.

What is Good Clinical Practice?

In the previous section, we discussed what clinical trials are and how different stakeholders such as investigators, sponsors, ethics committees and regulatory authorities work together to conduct a clinical study. But conducting a clinical trial involves more than simply following a study protocol. Because human participants are involved, the process must follow a set of ethical and scientific standards that ensure the safety, dignity and rights of participants. These standards are collectively called Good Clinical Practice (GCP).

Definition of Good Clinical Practice:

Good Clinical Practice refers to an internationally accepted set of ethical and scientific quality standards that must be followed while designing, conducting, recording and reporting clinical trials involving human participants.

The main objective of Good Clinical Practice is to ensure two important things:

1. Protection of the rights, safety and well-being of participants
2. Reliability and credibility of the data generated from the study

In simple words, Good Clinical Practice ensures that clinical research is conducted ethically, safely and scientifically.

If a clinical trial does not follow Good Clinical Practice, two major problems can occur. First, the participants may be exposed to unnecessary risk or harm. Second, the data generated from the study may not be reliable. If the data is unreliable, the results of the study cannot be trusted, and potentially unsafe treatment may reach patients.

Therefore, Good Clinical Practice protects both patients and science.

Origin of Good Clinical Practice:

The principles of Good Clinical Practice evolved over several decades as a response to unethical research practices that occurred in the past.

One of the most important historical events that influenced research ethics was the unethical medical experimentation conducted during the Second World War. This led to the development of the Nuremberg Code (1947) which emphasized voluntary consent of research participants.

Later, the Declaration of Helsinki, adopted by the World Medical Association in 1964, provided detailed ethical guidelines for research involving human participants.

Over the years, many countries developed their own clinical research regulations. However, as pharmaceutical research became global, it became necessary to have a common international standard.

This led to the development of International Council for Harmonization – Good Clinical Practice guidelines (ICH-GCP) in 1996. These guidelines harmonized clinical research standards across major regions such as the United States, Europe and Japan.

Today, most countries including India have adopted these principles while framing their own clinical trial regulations.

In India, Good Clinical Practice is enforced through regulatory authorities such as the Central Drugs Standard Control Organization (CDSCO) and through oversight by the respective Institutional Ethics Committees (IEC).

Why Good Clinical Practice is Important:

Clinical research involves testing interventions that are not yet fully proven to be safe or effective. Therefore, strict safeguards are required.

Good Clinical Practice ensures the following:

1. Protection of Participants

   The most important principle of GCP is that the well-being of the research participant takes priority over the interests of science and society. Participants must be protected from unnecessary risks. They must also be informed about:

a. The purpose of the study

b. The procedures involved

c. Possible benefits

d. Potential risks

Only after understanding these aspects should the participant or their legal guardian decide whether they want to participate.

2. Ethical Conduct of Research

Good Clinical Practice ensures that clinical trials are conducted ethically.

This includes:

a. Obtaining approval from an Institutional Ethics Committee

b. Ensuring informed consent

c. Avoiding exploitation of vulnerable populations

d. Maintaining participant confidentiality

Ethical oversight ensures that research participants are treated with dignity and respect.

3. Scientific Integrity

A clinical trial must not only be ethical but also scientifically sound. If a poorly designed study exposes participants to risk without the possibility of generating meaningful knowledge, the study itself becomes unethical.

Good Clinical Practice therefore requires:

a. A scientifically valid protocol

b. Appropriate sample size

c. Proper statistical planning

d. Qualified investigators

These ensure that the study produces reliable and meaningful results.

4. Data Quality and Transparency

Clinical trial data must be accurate and verifiable.

Good Clinical Practice requires:

a. Proper documentation of all study procedures

b. Maintenance of source records

c. Accurate reporting of outcomes

d. Transparent reporting of adverse events

This allows regulators and independent reviewers to verify the integrity of the study.

5. Accountability of Stakeholders

Clinical trials involve multiple stakeholders including investigators, sponsors, ethics committees and regulatory authorities.

Good Clinical Practice clearly defines the responsibilities of each stakeholder so that accountability is maintained throughout the study.

Core Principles of Good Clinical Practice:

Although Good Clinical Practice guidelines contain many detailed rules, they are all based on a few fundamental principles.

Let us briefly understand some of these principles.

1. Ethical Principles Must Be Followed

   Clinical trials must be conducted in accordance with ethical principles derived from international guidelines such as the Declaration of Helsinki.

2. Risk–Benefit Balance

   A clinical trial should only be conducted if the expected benefits justify the potential risks. If the risk becomes higher than anticipated during the study, appropriate action must be taken, including modifying or stopping the trial.

3. Rights and Safety of Participants are Paramount

   The interests of the participant must always come before the interests of science or commercial gain.

4. Informed Consent Is Essential

   Participation in a clinical trial must always be voluntary. Participants should be free to withdraw from the study at any time without affecting their regular medical care.

5. Qualified Investigators Must Conduct the Study

   Clinical trials must be conducted by investigators who are adequately trained and qualified. They must also have access to appropriate medical facilities and research infrastructure.

6. Accurate Documentation

   All clinical trial information must be recorded and stored in a way that allows accurate reporting, verification and interpretation. Proper documentation is a cornerstone of Good Clinical Practice.

7. Confidentiality of Participant Data

   Personal and medical information of participants must be protected. Only authorised individuals should have access to participant data.

Good Clinical Practice Is More Than Regulations:

Many people believe that Good Clinical Practice simply means following regulatory rules. However, this is only part of the concept.

Regulations describe the minimum standards required for conducting clinical research. But ethical responsibility often requires investigators and sponsors to go beyond these minimum requirements. For example, regulations may require reporting serious adverse events within a specified time period. However, an ethically responsible investigator will also carefully monitor participants and intervene early if a potential safety concern arises. Similarly, regulations may allow inclusion of certain vulnerable populations if appropriate safeguards are in place. But an investigator must still carefully consider whether the study is truly in the best interest of those participants.

Therefore, Good Clinical Practice should be viewed not merely as a regulatory requirement but as a professional and ethical commitment to protect participants and uphold scientific integrity.

Good Clinical Practice for Investigators:

Among all the stakeholders involved in a clinical trial, the investigator has the closest interaction with the study participant. The investigator examines the patient, explains the study, administers the investigational drug and monitors the patient for benefits and adverse effects. Because of this direct interaction, the investigator carries one of the greatest ethical responsibilities in clinical research.

Good Clinical Practice (GCP) provides clear guidance on how investigators should conduct clinical trials. These practices are intended to ensure that the rights, safety and well-being of participants are protected, while at the same time ensuring that the data generated from the study is scientifically reliable.

Let us understand what Good Clinical Practice means for investigators in practical terms.

1. **Adequate Qualification and Training:**

   Before agreeing to participate in a clinical trial, an investigator must ensure that he or she has the necessary qualifications and training to conduct the study.

   Clinical trials involve several procedures that are not part of routine clinical practice. These include:

   a. Understanding the study protocol

   b. Maintaining case record forms

   c. Reporting adverse events

   d. Following regulatory reporting timelines

   e. Maintaining drug accountability

   For this reason, investigators are expected to undergo Good Clinical Practice training before conducting clinical trials. The investigator should also be familiar with the scientific background of the study drug or device, which is usually provided in the Investigator's Brochure.

Accepting a clinical trial without understanding the study procedures or regulatory responsibilities may lead to errors that compromise both participant safety and data integrity.

2. **Understanding and Following the Study Protocol:**

The study protocol is the detailed written plan of the clinical trial. It describes the objectives of the study, eligibility criteria, treatment procedures, follow-up schedule and outcome measures.

One of the most important responsibilities of the investigator is to conduct the study strictly according to the approved protocol.

This includes:

a. Enrolling only participants who meet the inclusion criteria

b. Ensuring that exclusion criteria are respected

c. Administering the investigational product exactly as described

d. Performing required tests and assessments at the scheduled time

Failure to follow the protocol may result in protocol deviations or protocol violations, which can affect the scientific validity of the study.

However, there are situations where deviation from the protocol may be necessary to protect the safety of a participant. In such situations, the investigator may take appropriate medical decisions but must document and report the deviation to the sponsor and the Institutional Ethics Committee.

3. **Protecting the Rights and Safety of Participants:**

The most fundamental principle of Good Clinical Practice is that the rights, safety and well-being of research participants must take priority over the interests of science and society.

Investigators must therefore ensure that participants are not exposed to unnecessary risk.

This responsibility includes:

a. Careful assessment of eligibility before enrollment

b. Close monitoring of participants during the study

c. Prompt recognition of adverse events

Providing appropriate medical treatment when complications occur

If an investigator believes that continuing the study may harm the participant, the investigator must not hesitate to withdraw the participant from the study, even if this affects the study timeline. The investigator's duty as a doctor caring for a patient always comes before the role of a researcher.

4. **Proper Informed Consent Process:**

Obtaining informed consent is one of the most important responsibilities of the investigator. Informed consent is not merely obtaining a signature on a form. It is a process through which the participant understands the study and voluntarily decides whether to participate.

The investigator must explain:

a. The purpose of the study

b. The procedures involved

c. Potential benefits and possible risks

d. Alternative treatment options

e. The right to withdraw from the study at any time

The information should be provided in simple language that the participant can understand. In many situations, participants may require time to discuss the study with family members before deciding. The investigator should allow sufficient time for this decision-making process. In India, certain clinical trials also require audiovisual recording of the informed consent process, especially when vulnerable populations are involved (newborns, children, the elderly, mental illness, the critically ill, cancer patients etc)

5. **Accurate Documentation and Record Keeping:**

Good Clinical Practice places strong emphasis on accurate and complete documentation.

Investigators must maintain several types of records, including:

a. Case Record Forms (CRF)

b. Source documents (hospital records, laboratory reports

c. Adverse event records

d. Drug accountability logs

e. Participant follow-up records

These records allow the study to be verified and audited by sponsors, regulatory authorities and ethics committees. Incomplete or inaccurate documentation can lead to serious consequences, including rejection of study data by regulatory authorities.

Therefore, investigators should develop the habit of maintaining clear and timely documentation of all study-related activities.

6. **Reporting Adverse Events:**

During a clinical trial, participants may develop adverse events related to the investigational drug or procedure. Investigators must carefully monitor participants and document any adverse events.

Serious adverse events such as hospitalization, life-threatening complications or death must be reported to:

a. The sponsor

b. The Institutional Ethics Committee

c. Regulatory authorities (as required)

In many regulatory frameworks, serious adverse events must be reported within 24 hours of recognition.

Timely reporting allows safety signals to be identified early and appropriate action to be taken.

7. **Accountability of Investigational Product:**

Investigators are responsible for maintaining proper records of the investigational drug or device.

This includes:

a. Receiving the investigational product from the sponsor

b. Proper storage according to specified temperature conditions

c. Recording dispensing of the drug to participants

d. Maintaining records of unused or returned medication

This process is known as drug accountability. Proper accountability ensures that the investigational product is used only for study participants and prevents misuse or diversion.

8. **Communication with Ethics Committee and Sponsor:**

Investigators must maintain regular communication with both the Institutional Ethics Committee and the sponsor.

This includes:

a. Submitting periodic progress reports

b. Reporting serious adverse events

c. Informing about protocol deviations

d. Seeking approval for protocol amendments

e. Reporting completion of the study

This communication ensures transparency and allows oversight bodies to monitor the study effectively.

9. **Avoiding Conflict of Interest:**

Investigators must conduct research with professional integrity and independence. Financial or professional incentives should never influence decisions regarding participant enrollment, safety monitoring or reporting of results.

Investigators should disclose any potential conflicts of interest to the sponsor and the ethics committee. Transparency helps maintain public trust in clinical research.

10. **Going Beyond Regulatory Requirements:**

Ethical responsibility often requires investigators to go beyond these minimum requirements.

For example:

a. An investigator may decide to perform additional safety monitoring if early warning signs are detected.

b. An investigator may refuse to enroll vulnerable participants even if regulations technically permit it.

c. An investigator may halt recruitment temporarily if unexpected adverse events occur.

Such decisions reflect ethical judgment and professional responsibility, which are essential qualities of a good clinical investigator.

Good Clinical Practice for Sponsors:

In a clinical trial, the sponsor plays a central role in initiating, organizing and financing the research. While the investigator interacts directly with participants, the sponsor is responsible for ensuring that the entire clinical trial is designed and conducted according to ethical and scientific standards.

The sponsor may be a pharmaceutical company, biotechnology company, academic institution, government agency or a research organization. Regardless of who the sponsor is, Good Clinical Practice (GCP) requires that the sponsor ensures the clinical trial is conducted with scientific integrity and with full protection of participant safety.

The responsibilities of the sponsor begin even before the clinical trial starts and continue long after the study is completed.

Let us understand the principles of Good Clinical Practice for sponsors in detail.

1. **Designing a Scientifically Sound Study:**

   As already mentioned, one of the first responsibilities of the sponsor is to ensure that the clinical trial is scientifically valid.

   Before initiating a clinical trial, the sponsor must collect adequate information from:

   a. Laboratory studies

   b. Animal experiments

   c. Earlier phase clinical trials

   This information helps determine whether the intervention has sufficient evidence of safety and potential benefit to justify testing in humans.

   The sponsor must develop a well-designed study protocol that clearly describes study objectives, eligibility criteria, treatment procedures, outcome measures and statistical analysis plan.

2. **Selection of Qualified Investigators and Study Sites:**

   Sponsors must ensure that the clinical trial is conducted only at qualified research sites and by trained investigators.

   Before selecting a study site, the sponsor should evaluate investigator's clinical expertise, previous research experience, availability of research staff,adequacy of infrastructure,patient population relevant to the study.

   For example, a trial evaluating a treatment for pancreatic cancer should preferably be conducted in centers that treat a large number of such patients.

Sponsors must also ensure that investigators receive adequate training regarding the study protocol and Good Clinical Practice requirements.

3. **Regulatory and Ethics Approval:**

   Before starting a clinical trial, the sponsor must obtain approval from the relevant regulatory authorities and ethics committees. Regulatory authorities review the scientific data and determine whether the clinical trial can be safely conducted.

   Ethics committees review the ethical aspects of the study and the scientific validity of the study. In India, the sponsor must obtain approval from the Central Drugs Standard Control Organization (CDSCO) and also ensure that Institutional Ethics Committee (IEC) approval is obtained at every participating site. A clinical trial cannot begin until both regulatory and ethical approvals are granted.

4. **Providing the Investigational Product:**

   The sponsor is responsible for ensuring the quality and availability of the investigational product used in the study. This includes:

   a. Manufacturing the drug or device according to quality standards

   b. Proper labeling of the investigational product

   c. Packaging and transportation under appropriate conditions

   d. Supplying the product to study sites

   The sponsor must also maintain detailed records of investigational product accountability, ensuring that the drug is used only for study participants and stored under recommended conditions.

Poor quality or improperly stored investigational products can lead to unreliable study results and potential harm to participants.

5. **Monitoring the Clinical Trial:**

Good Clinical Practice requires that sponsors establish a monitoring system to ensure that the clinical trial is conducted according to the approved protocol.

Sponsors usually appoint trained professionals called clinical research monitors or clinical research associates (CRAs).

The responsibilities of monitors include:

a. Visiting study sites periodically

b. Verifying that participants meet eligibility criteria

c. Checking that informed consent has been properly obtained

d. Reviewing case record forms and source documents

e. Ensuring accurate data recording

Monitoring helps identify problems early and ensures that corrective actions are taken promptly.

6. **Ensuring Participant Safety:**

Protecting participant safety is one of the most important responsibilities of the sponsor. Sponsors must establish systems to collect and analyze safety information from all study sites.

This includes recording adverse events, reviewing serious adverse events, identifying safety signals across different study sites. If unexpected safety concerns arise, the sponsor must take appropriate action. This may include modifying the study protocol, temporarily suspending enrollment, informing investigators and regulatory authorities, terminating the trial if necessary

Some sponsors establish an independent Data and Safety Monitoring Board (DSMB) to periodically review safety data during large clinical trials.

7. **Reporting Safety Information to Regulators:**

Sponsors are responsible for reporting important safety information to regulatory authorities and ethics committees. Serious and unexpected adverse reactions must be reported according to regulatory timelines. Timely reporting ensures that regulators can monitor emerging safety concerns and intervene if necessary.

8. **Compensation and Insurance for Trial-Related Injury:**

Participants who volunteer for clinical trials may sometimes experience harm related to the investigational intervention. Good Clinical Practice requires that sponsors ensure medical care and financial compensation for participants who suffer trial-related injuries.

In India, sponsors must follow regulatory guidelines that require:

a. Free medical management of trial-related injury

b. Financial compensation for participants if the injury is directly related to the trial

c. Sponsors must also arrange insurance coverage to support these obligations.

This responsibility reflects the ethical principle that participants should not bear the burden of harm resulting from research.

9. **Ensuring Data Integrity and Transparency:**

Sponsors must ensure that the data generated from the clinical trial is accurate, reliable and transparent.

This involves:

a. Establishing data management systems

b. Conducting data verification

c. Performing statistical analysis according to the predefined plan

d. Maintaining study records for regulatory inspection

Sponsors must also ensure that study results are reported honestly, whether the results are positive or negative. Selective reporting or suppression of unfavorable data is considered unethical and undermines the credibility of scientific research.

10. **Responsibilities After Completion of the Trial:**

The responsibilities of the sponsor do not end when the clinical trial is completed. After completion of the study, the sponsor must analyze the study data carefully, prepare clinical study reports, submit results to regulatory authorities, publish findings in scientific literature when appropriate

If the investigational product receives regulatory approval, the sponsor must also support post-marketing surveillance studies to monitor long-term safety.

Going Beyond Regulatory Requirements

Responsible sponsors may establish independent safety monitoring boards even when not mandatory, provide additional participant support during the trial, ensure transparency in reporting both positive and negative results

Good Clinical Practice for Institutional Ethics Committees:

In clinical research, the Institutional Ethics Committee (IEC) plays a crucial role in protecting the rights, safety and well-being of participants. While investigators conduct the study and sponsors provide financial and logistical support, the ethics committee functions as an independent body that reviews and oversees the ethical aspects of the clinical trial.

Good Clinical Practice (GCP) requires that every clinical trial involving human participants must receive approval from an ethics committee before the study begins. The ethics committee must ensure that the study is ethically acceptable, scientifically reasonable and conducted with respect for human dignity.

Let us understand how Good Clinical Practice applies to the functioning of Institutional Ethics Committees.

1. **Independence of the Ethics Committee:**

   One of the fundamental requirements of Good Clinical Practice is that the ethics committee must function independently. The purpose of this independence is to ensure that the committee can make decisions based solely on ethical considerations, without pressure from investigators, sponsors or institutional authorities.

To maintain independence:

a. The Chairperson of the ethics committee is usually an external member who is not part of the institution conducting the research.

b. The committee includes members from different backgrounds, including medical, scientific, legal and social perspectives.

c. Decisions are taken collectively after discussion rather than by a single individual.

This diversity and independence ensure that the ethical review process is balanced and unbiased.

2. **Composition of the Ethics Committee:**

Good Clinical Practice guidelines emphasize that ethics committees must have diverse membership so that ethical decisions consider multiple perspectives.

A typical ethics committee includes:

a. A Chairperson, usually an external member

b. One or more clinicians, who can also be the member secretary

c. A basic medical scientist, often a pharmacologist, who can also be the member secretary

d. A legal expert, who is an external member

e. A social scientist or social worker, who is an external member

f. A layperson from the community, who is an external member

The member secretary, who is an internal member, coordinates the committee's activities, including meetings, the issuance of approval letters, regulatory submissions, and legal representation of the institutions in litigation.

The presence of both scientific and non-scientific members ensures that the ethical review considers not only technical scientific issues but also the social and ethical implications of the study.

For example, a clinician may assess the medical aspects of the protocol, while a social worker may identify potential exploitation of vulnerable populations.

3. **Ethical Review of the Study Protocol:**

Before a clinical trial begins, the ethics committee must carefully review the study protocol.

The committee evaluates several important aspects:

a. Whether the study has a clear scientific objective

b. Whether the study design is appropriate

c. Whether the risk–benefit balance is acceptable

d. Whether the participant population is appropriate

e. Whether vulnerable populations are being adequately protected

If the potential risks to participants are greater than the expected benefits, the ethics committee may reject the study or request modifications before approval. This review ensures that participants are not exposed to unnecessary risks.

4. Review of Informed Consent Documents:

Good Clinical Practice places great importance on the informed consent process, and ethics committees play a key role in ensuring that this process is ethically sound.

The ethics committee must review:

a. The participant information sheet

b. The informed consent form

c. The language used to explain the study

The information should be presented in a way that participants can easily understand.

The committee checks whether the consent document clearly explains:

a. The purpose of the study

b. Procedures involved

c. Possible benefits and risks

d. Participant rights

e. Compensation policies

In multilingual societies such as India, ethics committees also ensure that the consent documents are available in the local language so that participants fully understand the information provided.

5. Protecting Vulnerable Populations:

Some groups of participants may be particularly vulnerable to coercion or undue influence. These include children, pregnant women, economically disadvantaged individuals, mentally challenged persons, elderly individuals with limited decision-making capacity.

Good Clinical Practice requires ethics committees to take additional precautions when studies involve such vulnerable populations.

6. **Monitoring Ongoing Clinical Trials:**

The responsibility of the ethics committee does not end after granting approval to the study. Good Clinical Practice requires that ethics committees continuously monitor ongoing studies.

This monitoring includes:

a. Reviewing periodic progress reports from investigators

b. Reviewing reports of serious adverse events

c. Evaluating protocol deviations or violations

d. Conducting continuing review at regular intervals, usually annually

If new safety concerns arise during the study, the ethics committee may

a. Request modifications to the protocol

b. Temporarily suspend the study

c. Withdraw approval if participant safety is at risk

Continuous monitoring ensures that ethical oversight remains active throughout the study.

7. **Review of Serious Adverse Events:**

When serious adverse events occur during a clinical trial, investigators must report them to the ethics committee.

The ethics committee reviews these reports to determine:

a. Whether the adverse event is related to the investigational intervention

b. Whether participant safety is being adequately protected

c. Whether the study should continue without modification

In some situations, the ethics committee may recommend compensation for participants if the adverse event is related to the clinical trial. Such decisions help ensure that participants who suffer harm during research receive appropriate support.

8. **Maintaining Transparency and Documentation:**

Ethics committees must maintain proper documentation of all their activities.

This includes:

a. Records of protocol submissions

b. Minutes of ethics committee meetings

c. Decisions regarding approval or rejection of studies

d. Reports of adverse events and follow-up actions

Proper documentation ensures that the ethics committee's decisions are transparent and can be reviewed by regulatory authorities if necessary.

9. **Avoiding Conflict of Interest:**

Members of the ethics committee must avoid conflicts of interest. If a member is involved in a study being reviewed by the committee, that member must recuse themselves from the review process for that particular protocol. This ensures that the ethical review remains impartial and unbiased. Transparency regarding conflicts of interest is essential for maintaining public trust in the ethics review process.

10. Going Beyond Regulatory Requirements:

An ethics committee may request additional safety monitoring even when regulations do not require it, require simplified consent forms for participants with limited literacy, insist on additional safeguards for vulnerable participants.

Such actions reflect the committee's commitment to protecting research participants rather than merely fulfilling regulatory obligations.

Good Clinical Practice for Regulatory Authorities:

Regulatory authorities are government bodies that supervise clinical research and approve the use of drugs and medical devices in the general population. Their role is to ensure that clinical trials are conducted in accordance with scientific, ethical, and legal standards and that public health is protected.

Good Clinical Practice (GCP) applies not only to investigators and sponsors but also to regulators. Regulatory authorities must function with transparency, scientific competence and independence to maintain trust in the healthcare system.

Let us understand how Good Clinical Practice principles apply to the work of regulatory authorities.

1. Ensuring Scientific and Ethical Approval of Clinical Trials:

One of the primary responsibilities of regulatory authorities is to review clinical trial applications before a study begins. Sponsors must submit detailed information to the regulatory authority, including preclinical laboratory data, animal toxicity studies, earlier phase clinical trial results, manufacturing details of the investigational product and proposed clinical trial protocol

Regulators carefully evaluate whether the available evidence is sufficient to justify testing the intervention in humans.

The regulatory authority must ensure that the expected benefits justify the potential risks, the study design is scientifically sound, participant safety is adequately protected.

Only after this evaluation can permission be granted for the clinical trial to proceed.

2. **Establishing Clear Regulatory Guidelines:**

Regulatory authorities must develop and maintain clear rules that guide the conduct of clinical trials.

These regulations provide a framework for:

a. Ethical conduct of clinical research

b. Approval procedures for clinical trials

c. Safety monitoring requirements like web-portal for submission

d. Compensation for trial-related injury

e. Reporting of adverse events

Clear regulatory guidelines help investigators and sponsors understand the standards expected of them. These regulations are periodically updated to reflect evolving international standards and ethical considerations.

3. **Monitoring Compliance with Regulations:**

Approval of a clinical trial is not the end of regulatory oversight. Regulatory authorities must continue to monitor clinical trials to ensure that they are conducted according to approved protocols and regulatory requirements.

Monitoring activities may include:

a. Inspection of clinical trial sites

b. Review of study documentation

c. Examination of safety reports

d. Verification of compliance with Good Clinical Practice guidelines

During inspections, regulators may review:

a. Informed consent documentation

b. Case record forms

c. Investigational product accountability

d. Adverse event reports

If serious violations are identified, regulators have the authority to suspend or terminate the clinical trial.

4. **Ensuring Safety Reporting and Pharmacovigilance:**

Regulatory authorities must establish systems for monitoring the safety of investigational products. Sponsors and investigators are required to report serious adverse events to regulators within specified timelines.

Regulatory authorities analyze these reports to determine whether:

a. The adverse event is related to the investigational product

b. Similar safety concerns are occurring at multiple sites

c. Additional safety measures are required

If necessary, regulators may require:

a. Modifications to the study protocol

b. Additional safety monitoring

c. Temporary suspension of the trial

This system of safety reporting allows regulators to detect early signals of harm and protect participants.

5. **Approving Marketing Authorization:**

After successful completion of Phase III clinical trials, sponsors may apply for approval to market the drug or device.

Regulatory authorities evaluate extensive data before granting approval. This evaluation includes:

a. Evidence of clinical efficacy

b. Safety profile of the drug

c. Quality of manufacturing processes

d. Consistency of product formulation

Approval is granted only if the regulatory authority is satisfied that the benefits of the intervention outweigh the risks. In many cases, regulators may require additional studies or impose specific conditions before granting approval.

6. Post-Marketing Surveillance:

Even after a drug or medical device is approved, regulatory oversight continues.

Clinical trials often involve limited numbers of participants, and rare adverse events may not become apparent until the drug is used in a much larger population.

Regulatory authorities therefore require post-marketing surveillance, also known as pharmacovigilance.

This includes:

a. Monitoring reports of adverse drug reactions

b. Reviewing safety data from real-world clinical use

c. Conducting post-marketing studies when necessary

If new safety concerns arise, regulators may issue warnings, restrict the use of the drug or even withdraw the product from the market.

Several drugs have been withdrawn globally after rare but serious adverse effects were detected during post-marketing surveillance.

7. Going Beyond Minimum Regulation:

Regulators may require additional safety monitoring in high-risk trials, mandate registration of clinical trials in public registries, encourage publication of both positive and negative study results, promote transparency in clinical research.

These measures help strengthen the ethical and scientific framework of clinical research.

Final Thought:

Regulations play an essential role in governing clinical research. They establish the basic framework that ensures studies are conducted safely and responsibly. However, ethical responsibility in clinical research extends beyond regulatory compliance.

Investigators, sponsors, ethics committees and regulatory authorities must recognize that their primary responsibility is to protect the dignity, rights and safety of research participants. This responsibility requires thoughtful ethical judgment, professional integrity and a commitment to values that go beyond written rules.

Clinical research advances medical knowledge and improves patient care, but it must always be guided by the principle that human welfare takes precedence over scientific progress. By embracing ethical responsibility beyond regulations, researchers can ensure that clinical trials remain both scientifically valuable and ethically sound.

References:

1. International Council for Harmonisation (ICH).
2. *ICH E6(R2) Guideline for Good Clinical Practice.* Geneva: ICH; 2016.
3. Indian Council of Medical Research (ICMR).
4. *National Ethical Guidelines for Biomedical and Health Research Involving Human Participants.* New Delhi: ICMR; 2017.
5. Central Drugs Standard Control Organization (CDSCO).

6. *Good Clinical Practices for Clinical Research in India.* New Delhi: CDSCO; 2001.

7. World Medical Association.

8. *DeclarationofHelsinki:EthicalPrinciplesforMedicalResearch Involving Human Subjects.* JAMA. 2013;310(20):2191–2194.

Chapter 9

Ethical Issues in Study Designs and Statistics

Dr Gayathri T,
Department of Community Medicine, SRIHER, Chennai.
Gayathri.t@sriramachandra.edu.in

Abstract:

This chapter highlights key ethical issues in various study designs and statistical practices in biomedical research. It emphasizes that ethical research requires not only protection of participants through informed consent, confidentiality, and risk minimization, but also scientific validity through appropriate study design and analysis. Ethical concerns across case reports, cross-sectional, case–control, cohort studies, and randomized trials are discussed, along with issues such as data fabrication, misuse of statistics, and improper sample size. The chapter reinforces the importance of integrity, transparency, and responsible research conduct.

Keywords:

Research Ethics; Study Design; Statistics; Informed Consent; Confidentiality; Scientific Integrity; Data Fabrication; Sample Size

Objectives:

- Understand core ethical principles in research
- Identify ethical issues in different study designs
- Recognize unethical research practices
- Apply ethical principles in statistical analysis

Study designs are structured methods used in research for conducting a study scientifically valid and ethically sound. Different study designs are used depending on the objective of the study, the type of data required, and the feasibility of conducting the research. Common epidemiological study designs include descriptive studies such as case reports and case series, analytical studies such as cross-sectional, case-control and cohort studies and experimental studies such as randomized controlled trials (RCT). Each design has its own strengths, limitations, and ethical considerations that must be carefully addressed during the research process.

Ethical considerations vary across different study designs, but the core principles remain constant:

- Respect for autonomy
- Beneficence
- Non-maleficence
- Justice
- Scientific integrity
- Confidentiality
- Informed consent

1. What Makes a Study Unethical?

Before discussing the ethical issues related to individual study designs, it is important to understand that a study can be unethical even before it begins if it is scientifically not sound. A study may be considered unethical if it:

- Has a poor or inappropriate study design
- Is underpowered (i.e., has an inadequate sample size to answer the research question)
- Lacks clear objectives
- Uses inappropriate or incorrect statistical tests
- Is unlikely to produce valid, reliable, or meaningful results

Such studies waste funding and resources (exposing participants to unnecessary procedures) and weaken the credibility of the institution. Therefore, scientifically sound research must be considered ethical.

Case Report:

A case report describes a single patient with a rare condition, unusual presentation, or novel treatment outcome.

Ethical Concerns:

- Written informed consent from the patient is essential before publication.
- Strict confidentiality must be maintained.
- Identifiers such as name, hospital number, or address must be removed.
- Clinical photographs must not reveal identity.

Because rare cases are easily identifiable, extra care must be taken to protect patient privacy.

Case Series:

A case series describes multiple patients with a similar condition or treatment outcome, without a control group.

Ethical Concerns:

- Consent must be obtained from all included patients.
- Data must be reported honestly without selective inclusion of only favorable cases.
- Confidentiality must be strictly maintained.

Selective reporting or exaggeration of outcomes is unethical.

Cross-Sectional Studies:

A cross-sectional study assesses both exposure and outcome at a single point in time, providing a snapshot of the characteristics of a population.

Ethical Concerns:

Although cross-sectional studies are generally considered low risk, they still raise important ethical issues:

- **Sensitive questions:** Topics such as mental health, sexual behaviour, substance use, income, and domestic violence may cause discomfort.
- **Minimal risk:** Questionnaires must not cause psychological distress.
- **Sampling fairness:** No group should be excluded without scientific justification. Participation must be voluntary.

- **Confidentiality:** Responses must remain anonymous to prevent stigma or discrimination.

Many studies conducted among school children are cross-sectional in nature, as they often involve surveys that collect information on health behaviours, lifestyle factors, or psycho social issues at a single point in time. Although cross-sectional studies are relatively simple to conduct, special ethical considerations are required when the participants are minors. Therefore, research involving school students must follow strict ethical guidelines, including obtaining appropriate administrative permissions, parental consent, and ensuring the protection of the child's welfare and confidentiality.

1. Administrative Approvals:

When research is conducted in schools, permission from relevant educational authorities is required in addition to institutional ethical approval. The required approvals may vary depending on the type of school.

2. Parental Consent and Assent:

Parental consent must be obtained from parents or legal guardians before including children (<18 yrs)in the study. In addition to parental consent, written assent form must be obtained from children with more than 11 years and oral assent form for children between 7 and 11 years. For children with less than 7 years, parental consent alone is enough.

3. Research on Sensitive Topics:

Sensitive topics such as physical abuse require special care and ethical consideration during research. Parents should be made aware through the consent form that any disclosure of abuse could be reported to the relevant authorities or the police.

Case–Control Studies:

A case–control study involves comparing people who have a specific disease (cases) with those who do not have the disease (controls) in order to identify possible factors associated with the condition.

Ethical Concerns:

- **Voluntary participation:** Controls must not feel pressured to participate.
- **Recall bias stress:** Participants may experience emotional stress while recalling past trauma, accidents, or illness.
- **Sensitive exposure history:** Smoking, alcohol use, and sexual history must be handled confidentially.
- **Selection of Controls:** Controls must be selected fairly and without bias. It is unethical to select controls in a way that if they misrepresents the comparison group.

  Leads to misleading or invalid conclusions.

Ethical Issues in Cohort Studies:

Cohort studies follow exposed and unexposed individuals over time to observe outcomes.

Ethical Concerns:

- **Participant burden:** Multiple visits and repeated assessments may cause inconvenience, especially for individuals without exposure.

- **Repeated tests:** Blood tests, imaging, and radiological investigations carry risk. Controls must not be unnecessarily exposed to radiation solely for comparison purposes.
- **Risk–benefit balance:** Procedures must be justified scientifically.Participants should not undergo invasive or risky procedures unless it is clearly necessary.

Randomized Controlled Trials (RCT):

A randomized controlled trial involves random allocation of participants into an intervention group and a control group in order to evaluate the effectiveness of a treatment or intervention.

Ethical Concerns:

Randomization is a fundamental feature of randomized controlled trials, as it helps ensure that participants are allocated to different study groups purely by chance. Randomization should be conducted using appropriate methods, such as computer generated random sequences to prevent manipulation or selection bias.

- **Trial Registration :** Clinical trials should be registered in the Clinical Trials Registry of India before enrolling participants
- **Use of placebo :** Ethical only when no proven effective treatment exists.
- **Stopping rules:** If the intervention is clearly harmful, the trial must be stopped early.
- **Risk minimization:** Risks must be reasonable compared to potential benefits.
- Withholding standard care

- Unnecessary invasive procedures
- High-risk interventions with little scientific value
- Exposing participants to harm without safeguards

Ethical Concern When Harm Is Already Established:

For instance, if many studies have already been mentioned that a particular drug or intervention produces some serious adverse events, again doing the study with the same intervention is unethical.Therefore, review of literature is must for any scientific research.

Whether the study is cross-sectional, case–control, cohort, experimental, or record-based, the researcher has a moral responsibility to protect participants, use resources wisely, and uphold academic integrity.

Ethical issues in statistics:

Ethical research is not only limited to obtaining consent forms, confidentiality, protection, risk minimization, scientifically sound design and continues through fair participant selection(sampling) and responsible reporting.

Statistics plays a crucial role in scientific research in order to design studies, calculate sample size, analyze data and interpret results. Statistical findings influence medical practice, public health policies, and scientific knowledge. Because of this impact, statistics must be used responsibly and ethically.

Ethical issues in statistics arise when data are manipulated, misinterpreted, selectively reported, or analyzed using inappropriate methods. Ethical statistical practice ensures honesty, transparency and reliability in research.

1. Honesty in Data Collection and Reporting:

Ethical use of research questionnaires/ instruments

Researchers must ensure the ethical use of research instruments. When an existing questionnaire or instrument is used, researchers should verify whether it is freely available or, if required, obtain permission from the original author. Using a copyrighted questionnaire without permission may violate ethical standards. If a researcher develops a new questionnaire for the study, it should undergo appropriate validation and reliability testing before being used for data collection.

Data should be collected and reported accurately by the researchers without any modification of the results. Fabrication or falsification of data is regarded as a major violation of research ethics.

2. Data Fabrication and Falsification:

Fabrication involves generating false data that do not exist in reality. Falsification occurs when researchers change or distort data to support a particular conclusion. Both practices are unethical and damage scientific credibility.

3. Selective Reporting and P-Hacking:

Researchers explore several analyses with different statistical methods and selectively report the significant results; this practice is known as p-hacking.

4. Misuse of Statistical Tests:

Selecting the wrong statistical method may produce invalid conclusions.

Common problems include:

- Applying unsuitable statistical tests
- Ignoring the assumptions required for statistical methods
- Failing to control or adjust for confounding variables
- Confusing statistical significance with clinical significance
- Not adjusting the analysis when several statistical tests are performed.

Incorrect analysis may lead to wrong clinical recommendations.

Ethical Issues in Sample Size:

An ethically conducted study must determine an appropriate sample size through proper statistical calculation to get valid results by minimizing unnecessary participant involvement.

Under powered studies: If the sample size is too small, the study may not detect a real effect. This exposes participants to research without generating meaningful or valid results, which is ethically unacceptable.

Excessively large sample size: Recruiting more participants than necessary exposes additional individuals to potential risks, inconvenience, or procedures without scientific justification.

Wastage of resources: An inappropriate sample size can lead to unnecessary funding, time and participant effort.

Conclusion:

Ethical research is not only limited to obtaining consent forms,confidentiality protection, risk minimization, it also includes a scientifically sound design, honest data collection, appropriate statistical analysis, transparent reporting and responsible interpretation. When study design and statistics are used responsibly, this may leads to reliable evidence-based decision-making in medicine and public health.

References:

1. Indian Council of Medical Research. National Ethical Guidelines for Biomedical and Health Research Involving Human Participants. New Delhi: ICMR; 2017.

2. World Medical Association. World Medical Association Declaration of Helsinki: Ethical Principles for Medical Research Involving Human Subjects. JAMA. 2013;310(20):2191–2194. doi:10.1001/jama.2013.281053

Chapter 10

Informed Consent

Dr Anupma Jyoti Kindo MD
Professor in the Department of Microbiology Member
Secretary Ethics Committee
Email ID anupmalakra@gmail.com

Abstract:

Informed consent is a fundamental ethical and legal principle in medicine and research, safeguarding patient autonomy by requiring voluntary agreement based on full disclosure of risks, benefits, and alternatives. Emerging from 20th- century U.S. cases like Schloendorff vs. Society of New York Hospital (1914), which affirmed bodily inviolability, and Salgo vs. Stanford (1957), which coined the term, it gained urgency post-World War II via the Nuremberg Code (1947) mandating voluntary participation in experiments. Key milestones include the Declaration of Helsinki (1964), revelations of unethical trials like Tuskegee (1972), and the Belmont Report (1979), establishing respect for persons, beneficence, and justice. Today, codified in regulations like the U.S. Common Rule, it demands comprehension, capacity, and voluntariness, yet faces challenges from complex forms, vulnerable populations, and innovations like digital consent. This chapter elucidates its evolution, elements, applications, and future directions for ethical practice.

Objectives:

- Outline the legal and ethical origins of informed consent
- Examine key milestones shaping its global standards
- Define core components and regulatory frameworks
- Analyze core elements, applications and contemporary challenges

Historical and Guideline Foundations:

Legal origins:

The term "Informed Consent" originated in the 1957 Salgo vs. Leland Stanford Jr. university Board of Trustees case, where a patient suffered paralysis from an undisclosed procedure risk, mandating physicians to disclose material hazards.

Research Ethics Reforms (1947-1979):

Nazi experiments led to the 1947 Nuremberg Code, mandating voluntary consent with full disclosure of risks, purpose, and withdrawal rights as its first principle.

The 1964 Declaration of Helsinki, Henry Beecher's 1966 exposé on unethical U.S. trials, the 1972 Tuskegee Syphilis Study revelation, and the 1979 Belmont Report (emphasizing information, comprehension and voluntariness) shaped modern standards.

Codification and Modern Standards:

U.S. common rule requires disclosure of purpose, risks, benefits, alternatives and voluntariness; 2018 updates added a 'key information' summary for comprehension. Elements include disclosure, capacity (understanding/ appreciation/ reasoning), and voluntariness (no coercion); waivers apply in emergencies or minimal-risk research.

Challenges and Innovations: Long forms hinder comprehension; solutions include tiered disclosures, videos and dynamic consent models.

Salgo vs. Leland Stanford Jr. University Board of Trustees (1957):

This case shifted focus from simple consent (Schloendorff) to informed consent, requiring disclosure od procedure-specific risks, benefits, and alternatives. It underpins modern standards like the U.S. Common rule mandating summaries of key information (purpose, risks, benefits, and voluntariness).

The Nuremberg Code of 1947:

The Nuremberg Code of 1947 emerged from the Doctor's Trial at the Nuremberg Military Tribunals, prosecuting Nazi physicians for war crimes involving inhumane experiments on concentration camp prisoners during World War II.

Nuremberg Military Tribunal's decision in the case of the United States vs Karl Brandt et al. includes what is now called the Nuremberg Code, a ten-point statement delimiting permissible medical experimentation is justified only if its results benefit society and it is carried out in accord with basic principles that "satisfy moral, ethical, and legal concepts."

--"Permissible Medical Experiments." Trials of War Criminals before the Nuremberg Military Tribunals under Control Council Law No. 10 Nuremberg October 1946- April 1949, Washington US Government Printing Office (n.d.), vol. 2., pp.181-182.

The 10-point statement:

1. The human subject's voluntary consent is important. This means that the individual in question must have the legal capacity to give consent, be in a position that allows him to exercise his free will without the interference of any element of force, fraud, deceit, duress, overreach, or other hidden form of constraint or coercion, and possess adequate knowledge and comprehension of the relevant subject matter to enable him to make an informed and understanding decision. This latter requirement stipulates that the experimental subject must be informed of the nature, duration, and purpose of the experiment; the method and means by which it is to be conducted; all inconveniences and hazards that are reasonably to be expected; and any potential effects on his health or person that may result from his participation in the experiment before accepting an affirmative decision.

   Each person who initiates, oversees, or participates in the experiment bears the obligation and responsibility for determining the quality of the consent. It is a personal obligation and responsibility that cannot be transferred to another person without consequence.

2. The experiment should produce results that are beneficial to society, unobtainable through alternative research techniques, and not haphazard or superfluous.

3. The experiment should be planned so that the expected outcomes would support the experiment's execution, based on the findings of animal testing and an understanding of the natural history of the illness or other issue being studied.

4. The experiment should be carried out in a way that prevents any needless harm or suffering to the body or mind.
5. With the possible exception of studies in which the experimental physicians are also subjects, no experiment should be carried out if there is an a priori cause to assume that death or a disabling damage will occur.
6. The level of risk should never be greater than what is determined by the humanitarian significance of the issue that the experiment is intended to address.
7. To safeguard the experimental subject from even remote risks of damage, impairment, or death, proper preparations should be made and sufficient facilities should be supplied.
8. Only those with scientific qualifications should carry out the experiment. Those who perform or participate in the experiment should be held to the highest standards of skill and caution throughout the entire process.
9. The human subject shall have the freedom to stop the experiment at any time if he reaches a point in his physical or mental state where he believes it is impossible to continue.
10. Throughout the experiment, the responsible scientist must be ready to end it at any point if he has good reason to believe—in the exercise of the good faith, superior skill, and careful judgment required by him—that continuing the experiment will likely cause harm, disability, or death to the experimental subject.

The Declaration of Helsinki (1964, amended through 2013):

The Declaration of Helsinki, adopted in 1964 by the World Medical Association (WMA) in Helsinki, Finland, builds on the Nuremberg Code to provide ethical guidelines for medical research involving human subjects. It sets out ethical principles for medical research involving human participants, data, or material, emphasizing that subject welfare must take precedence over science. Key requirements include informed consent, risk assessment, and independent ethical review.

Key aspects of the Declaration include:

- Fundamental Principle: The health and rights of research participants take precedence over the interests of science and society.
- Informed Consent: Participation must be voluntary, and subjects must be fully informed of risks, benefits, and the right to withdraw.
- Ethical Review: Research protocols must be submitted to an independent, qualified ethics committee for approval before starting.
- Vulnerable groups: Special protections are required for populations that are vulnerable or unable to give consent.
- Updates: The Declaration is a "living document" that is revised periodically, with a new version adopted in October 2024 to address modern challenges.
- Scope: While not legally binding, it is widely adopted into national legislation and international regulations.

National bodies like ICMR require Helsinki compliance in ethics protocols enforcing independent review, ongoing monitoring, and community engagement.

The Belmont Report (1979):

Key aspects of the Belmont Report:

Background: The Belmont Report, published in 1979 by the U.S. National Commission for the Protection of Human Subjects of Biomedical and Behavioral Research, established foundational ethical principles for research involving human subjects, responding to scandals like the Tuskegee Syphilis Study.

Three Core Principles:

Respect for Persons: Acknowledging autonomy and protecting individuals with diminished autonomy, requiring informed consent.

Beneficence: Maximising benefits and minimising risks through systematic risk-benefit assessment; "Do no harm" while ensuring research justifies any risks.

Justice: Ensuring fairness in the distribution of research burdens and benefits. The five core elements of informed consent are Competence (ability to decide), Disclosure (providing all relevant info), Understanding (comprehending the info), Voluntariness (free form coercion), and Consent/ Authorization (agreement to proceed). These ensure a person can make an autonomous, educated decision about participating in a medical procedure or research study.

Breakdown of each element:

- **Competence/ Capacity:** The individual must have the mental ability to understand the information and make a reasoned decision.
- **Disclosure:** Providers must give clear, comprehensive information about the treatment/ study, including risks, benefits, alternatives, and costs.
- **Understanding:** The patient must comprehend the disclosed information, not just hear it.
- **Voluntariness:** The decision to consent must be made freely, without pressure, manipulation, or coercion.
- **Consent/Authorisation:** The person must actively agree to the proposed action, often through a signature, though it can be verbal.

Other key aspects often included are the right to withdraw, confidentiality, and specifics about the procedures involved, ensuring a thorough and ethical process.

Applications:

- Informed Consent: Subjects must be given information, understand it and voluntarily participate.
- Assessment of Risks and Benefits: A systematic assessment of potential harms versus benefits.
- Selection if Subjects: Fair procedures to ensure vulnerable populations are not exploited.
- Distinction: The report distinguishes between research (designed to develop knowledge) and practice (designed to enhance an individual's wellbeing).

- The principles outlined in the report are central to modern institutional review boards (IRBs) and federal regulations (45CFR 46) governing research ethics.
- The informed consent requires respect for persons via voluntary entry with adequate information in human subject research; Informed consent protects the individual's freedom of choice and respects the individual's autonomy.

Core Principles of Informed Consent:

The basic principle of informed consent, which ensures that participants choose to take part in research or treatment voluntarily and with information, is respect for individual autonomy. From the initial engagement through the study, information must be given in a language suitable for the participant's comprehension level.

Investigators must verify understanding, allow unrestricted questions, consider cultural factors (e.g., community leader permission not substituting individual consent), renew consent for new information or procedure changes, ensure voluntarism without coercion/ inducement, prioritize written consent (signed by subject or guardian), and permit oral consent for minimal-risk studies with IEC approval. Drugs and Cosmetics Rules (5th Amendment, 2015) mandate audio-visual recording for vulnerable subjects in new chemical entity trials (audio only for Anti- HIV/ Anti-leprosy).

Basic Information Requirements:

Consent documents in clinical research consist of a Participant Information Sheet (PIS) and an Informed Consent Form (ICF), which must be provided to participants as copies after consent is obtained. The signing process requires participants to sign or thumb-print the documents only after fully understanding the information, with investigators co-signing and dating them. Essential elements include details of the Principal Investigator (PI) or sponsor, a free invitation to participate, study purpose, procedures (including randomisation), duration, number of visits, and any compensation. The result disclosure and data access, predictable risks or discomforts, potential benefits, availability of alternative effective treatments, patent benefits, provisions for free treatment, compensation, and insurance for injuries related to research, privacy and confidentiality measures (with stigma counselling if applicable), use of biological materials or data, publication plans, and statements on placebo use or therapeutic failure in accordance with Drugs Rules are additional essential components.

Further requirements encompass Institutional Ethics Committee (IEC) approval details, funding information, and contact details for relevant helplines such as those for multiple sclerosis (MS). These elements ensure participants are fully informed, enabling voluntary and ethical involvement in the study.

Informed Consent Form Template:

The template includes study title/number, subject initials/ name/age, statements confirming understanding/voluntary participation/record access/agreement to join, signatures/ thumb impressions of subject/LAR/investigator/witness with dates and names. This standard format ensures clarity and accountability in the consent process.

An informed consent form is a crucial document and process ensuring participants fully understand a study's purpose, procedures, risks, and benefits before voluntarily agreeing to join. It acts as a written record of this communication, outlining voluntary participation, data confidentiality, and the right to withdraw without penalty.

Key Components of an Informed Consent Form:

- **Study Details:** Clearly stated purpose, duration, and specific procedures involved.
- **Risks & Benefits:** Honest explanation of potential side effects, discomforts, or unknown risks.
- **Voluntary Participation:** Explicit statement that participation is voluntary and refusal will not affect care.
- **Confidentiality:** How personal data or biological samples will be protected.
- **Contact Information:** Names and details of researchers for questions.
- **Signature Page:** Dated signatures from the participant (or legal representative) and the researcher

Assent Form:

An assent form is a document, often used for children (typically ages 7–17) or individuals with impaired decision-making capacity, to obtain their affirmative agreement to participate in research, distinct from legal parental/guardian consent. It explains the study in simple, age-appropriate language.

Guidelines for Assent:

- **Age Appropriateness:** For children 7–11, verbal or simplified written assent is used. For children 12–17, written assent is usually required.
- **Process:** The form should be read to or reviewed with the child in a way they understand.
- **Consent:** Assent must be obtained *in addition* to the informed consent of a parent or legal guardian.
- **Voluntary:** The child›s refusal to sign should be respected, even if the parent has given consent.

Sample Assent Structure:

i. Title of Project

ii. Introduction: My name is (name) and I am studying (topic)

iii. Why are we doing this?

iv. What will I do?

v. Do I have to do this? (Voluntary participation statement)

Essential Guidelines:

- Language: Must be simple, easy to understand, and ideally in the participant's native language.
- Process: It is more than just a signature; it is a dialogue to ensure understanding.
- Living Document: Should be updated if new information arises during the trial

- Waiver of Informed Consent: A waiver of informed consent is an Institutional Review Board (IRB) approved exception allowing research to proceed without obtaining formal, written consent from participants. It is granted only for studies with minimal risk, such as retrospective chart reviews or anonymous surveys, where obtaining consent is impractical and participant rights are not compromised. To qualify for a waiver of informed consent, the research must meet specific ethical and regulatory criteria.
- Minimal risk: The research involves no more than minimal risk to the participant's welfare or privacy.
- Practicability: The research could not reasonably be performed without the waiver (e.g., impossible to locate participants for a large, old database study).
- No Adverse Effects: The waiver will not adversely affect the rights and welfare of the subjects.
- Inform Participants: Whenever appropriate, participants will be provided with additional information after the participation (e.g., debriefing).

Common Scenarios for Waivers:

- **Retrospective Chart Review:** Analysing medical records without direct patient contact.
- **Anonymous Data/ Bio-specimens:** Using de-identified data or stored samples.
- **Emergency Research:** Situations where obtaining consent is time-critical and not possible, often requiring urgent intervention.

Waiver of Consent vs. Waiver of Documentation:

- **Waiver of Consent:** The entire process of informing the patient and getting their permission is waived.
- **Waiver of Documentation:** The researcher still informs the participant (verbal consent) but does not require a signature, usually because the signature is the only link to confidentiality.

Principal Investigators cannot unilaterally waive consent; IECs may approve partial/ full waivers for minimal risk research impracticable otherwise, de-identified retrospective stuies, anonymized samples/ data, public-domain data, surveillance/ evaluation. IEC decisions prioritize participant rights and feasibility.

Specific Situations:

- Limited capacity individuals
- Young children (7-18years): Require parental/LAR consent + Oral assent (7-12years) or written assent (12+ years)
- Incompetents: Require guardian permission; no inducements beyond expenses
- Biological materials in trials
- Use separate sections/ forms for consent (blanket, tiered, or specific)
- Clinical care records/ specimens
- Need IEC approval for minimal risk, rights-respecting research where consent is impracticable
- Secondary use

- Must align with original consent or ensure anonymity
- Genetic research
- Demands stringent consent, choices for result/ incidental finding disclosure, and family/ community consents.
- Emergencies (e.g., stroke)
- Require prior IEC approval, early consent from at-risk groups, relative proxy consent, post-inclusion re-consent, and discontinuation if refusal occurs.

Templates are available in the WHO Ethics Review Committee website:

- Informed consent for clinical studies
- Consent for storage and future use of unused samples
- Informed consent for qualitative studies
- Informed assent for children/ minors
- Informed parental consent for research involving children (Qualitative)
- Informed parental consent research involving children (Clinical)

The logo of the Institution must be used on the ICF and not the WHO logo.

References:

1. 1.https://www.fda.gov › search-fda-guidance-documents
2. ICMR - Bioethics Unit https://ethics.ncdirindia.org
3. Indian Council of Medical Research: https://www.icmr.gov.in › uploads › Guidelines

Chapter 11

Serious Adverse Drug Events (SAEs) And Ethical Reporting

Dr. D. Anusha
Professor, Department of Pharmacology
SRMC&RI
SRIHER, Porur, Chennai-600116
Email – drdanusha@gmail.com

Abstract:

Serious Adverse Drug Events (SAEs) represent the most severe outcomes associated with drug therapy and remain a major concern in modern healthcare. Despite extensive preclinical testing and phased clinical trials, medicines may still produce adverse effects when used in diverse populations under real-world conditions. SAEs include events that result in death, life-threatening conditions, hospitalization, persistent disability, congenital anomalies, or other medically significant outcomes requiring intervention. These events contribute significantly to patient morbidity, mortality, prolonged hospital stays, and increased healthcare costs worldwide.

Pharmacovigilance systems play a critical role in identifying, assessing, and preventing serious adverse drug events. However, underreporting remains a major challenge due to factors such as lack of awareness, uncertainty in causality assessment, time constraints, and fear of legal consequences. Ethical reporting of SAEs is therefore essential to ensure early detection of drug safety signals and to protect patients from preventable harm. The ethical framework governing SAE reporting is grounded in the principles of beneficence, non-maleficence, autonomy, justice, transparency, and professional integrity.

Multiple stakeholders—including healthcare professionals, clinical investigators, pharmaceutical industries, and regulatory authorities—share responsibility for accurate and timely reporting of SAEs. Strengthening pharmacovigilance systems through education, simplified reporting mechanisms, supportive institutional policies, and international collaboration can significantly improve reporting practices.

In conclusion, ethical and transparent reporting of serious adverse drug events is essential for safeguarding patient safety, improving drug regulation, and maintaining public trust in healthcare systems. Continuous efforts to enhance awareness, regulatory compliance, and technological innovations will further strengthen global pharmacovigilance and responsible drug use.

Introduction:

Medicines are among the most powerful tools in modern healthcare, contributing significantly to disease prevention, treatment, and improved quality of life. Despite rigorous preclinical research and phased clinical trials, no medicinal product can be considered entirely free from risk. Adverse drug events remain an inevitable consequence of pharmacotherapy, particularly when drugs are used in diverse populations under real-world conditions.

Among all adverse outcomes related to drug use, Serious Adverse Drug Events (SAEs) represent the most critical category due to their potential to cause death, life-threatening conditions, hospitalisation, permanent disability, or congenital anomalies. The growing complexity of drug therapy, polypharmacy, and the introduction of novel biological and targeted therapies have further increased the importance of continuous drug safety monitoring.

Ethical reporting of SAEs forms the backbone of pharmacovigilance systems worldwide. It ensures early detection of safety signals, protects patients from preventable harm, and maintains public confidence in healthcare systems. This chapter-style discussion explores the scientific, regulatory, and ethical dimensions of serious adverse drug events and emphasizes the moral obligation of transparent and timely reporting.

Concept and Definition of Serious Adverse Drug Events:

Serious Adverse Event is defined as any undesirable medical occurrence associated with the use of a medicinal product that results in outcomes such as death, life-threatening conditions, hospitalisation, or prolongation of hospitalisation, persistent disability, congenital anomaly, or any medically significant condition requiring intervention.

International regulatory bodies, including the International Council for Harmonisation, have standardised the definition of SAEs to ensure uniformity in reporting and evaluation across countries. The term “serious” refers to the outcome or consequence of the event rather than its intensity. It’s important to know how to differentiate between adverse events, adverse drug reactions, and serious adverse events. While an adverse effect may not necessarily have a causal relationship with a drug, an adverse drug reaction implies a reasonable association. They are distinguished by their occurrence, frequency, severity, and regulatory significance, requiring expedited reporting and a thorough causality assessment.

Epidemiology and Burden of Saes:

Serious adverse drug events constitute a major public health concern globally. Studies published in peer-reviewed journals indicate that a substantial proportion of hospital admissions and in-hospital complications are attributable to drug-related harm. SAEs significantly increase healthcare costs, length of hospital stay, and patient morbidity and mortality.

Vulnerable populations such as the elderly, paediatric patients, pregnant women, and individuals with chronic illnesses are particularly susceptible. Polypharmacy, age-related physiological changes, and comorbidities further elevate the risk of serious adverse outcomes.

Though their impact, SAEs are widely underreported. Literature consistently demonstrates that only a fraction of serious drug reactions are captured by spontaneous reporting systems. This underreporting delays regulatory action and compromises patient safety, highlighting the ethical imperative for improved reporting practices.

Classification of Serious Adverse Drug Events:

Classification of serious adverse drug events is essential for systematic evaluation, regulatory decision-making, and ethical reporting. Proper categorisation enables healthcare professionals, researchers, and regulators to assess severity, causality, and urgency of intervention. Multiple classification systems are used in pharmacovigilance literature to ensure consistency and clarity.

Classification Based on Clinical Outcome:

Based on clinical consequences, SAEs are categorised into distinct outcome-based groups. Fatal adverse drug events represent the most severe form and demand immediate investigation and regulatory action. Life-threatening adverse events are those in which the patient was at immediate risk of death at the time of the event, even if death did not occur.

International regulatory guidelines (such as ICH-GCP) define a Serious Adverse Event (SAE) as any unfavourable medical event that:

- Enables death
- Is it potentially fatal?
- Needs an inpatient stay or an extension of an already-existing hospital stay
- Causes a major or persistent handicap or infirmity
- Results in a birth deformity or congenital abnormality
- Needs action to stop irreversible harm or impairment It's critical to distinguish between: Any negative medical event is referred to as an adverse event (AE).

- An adverse drug reaction, also called an ADR, is an adverse event (AE) that is caused by a medication.
- SAE is determined by the severity of the consequence rather than by causality.

It is important to remember that all SAEs are adverse events, but not all adverse events are SAEs

A "Life Threatening Adverse Drug Experience" defined as

Any adverse experience that places the subject, in the view of the investigator, at immediate risk of death from the reaction as it occurred, or it is suspected that the use or continued use of the product would result in the patient's death.

"Congenital Anomaly" defined as exposure to a medical product prior to conception or during pregnancy resulting in an adverse outcome in the child.

Why SAEs matter:

They are critical safety signals in both clinical trials and post-marketing surveillance. Identifying SAEs early helps regulators, healthcare providers, and pharmaceutical companies protect patients and adjust treatment guidelines. Hospitalisation-related SAEs include both events that cause new hospital admissions and those that prolong existing hospital stays. These events significantly increase healthcare burden and costs. Disability-related SAEs involve persistent or significant impairment of physical or mental functioning, often leading to long-term dependence and reduced quality of life. Congenital anomalies or birth defects associated with drug exposure during pregnancy constitute a unique and ethically sensitive category requiring special surveillance.

SAEs are commonly categorised according to their clinical consequences:

- Fatal adverse drug events
- Life-threatening reactions
- Events requiring hospitalisation or prolongation of hospital stay
- Events resulting in permanent disability
- Congenital anomalies or birth defects

Each category carries specific implications for clinical management and regulatory action.

Classification Based on Predictability:

SAEs may be classified as expected or unexpected. Expected SAEs are consistent with known safety information, whereas unexpected SAEs differ in nature or severity from existing data. Unexpected SAEs are particularly important for signal detection and regulatory review.

SAEs are also classified as expected or unexpected based on prior safety information. Expected SAEs are consistent with known pharmacological properties and are documented in the product label or investigator brochure. Unexpected SAEs differ in nature, severity, or frequency from existing data and are of high regulatory importance.

Unexpected SAEs often serve as early warning signals for previously unidentified risks. Ethical concerns arise when such events are not promptly reported, as delayed recognition may expose larger populations to preventable harm.

Classification Based on Causality:

Causality assessment aids in evaluating the probability that a drug was responsible for an event. While it can be challenging, conducting a transparent causality assessment is ethically crucial to guarantee the reliability of pharmacovigilance data. Because establishing causality conclusively can be difficult, structured methods are employed to categorize serious adverse events (SAEs) as:

Definitely related

Probably related

Possibly related

Unlikely related

Unrelated

Ethical reporting mandates that all SAEs, including those that are uncertain or suspected, be reported, since causality assessments become more accurate as data accumulates from multiple reports

Causes and Mechanisms of Saes:

Serious adverse drug events arise from a complex interaction of drug-related, patient-related, and system-related factors. Drug characteristics such as narrow therapeutic index, high potency, and complex metabolism increase the likelihood of serious reactions. Drug–drug and drug–food interactions are major contributors, particularly in patients receiving multiple medications.

Patient-specific factors include age, genetic variations, organ dysfunction, pregnancy, and immune status. Healthcare system failures such as prescribing errors, inadequate monitoring, poor communication, and lack of patient education further contribute to preventable SAEs.

Drug-Related Factors:

Drug-related factors include pharmacokinetic and pharmacodynamic properties. Drugs with a narrow therapeutic index pose a higher risk of serious toxicity. Errors in dose calculation, formulation changes, or bioavailability can easily lead to life-threatening outcomes.

Drug–drug interactions are a major cause of SAEs, particularly in patients receiving multiple medications. Enzyme inhibition or induction may result in toxic drug levels or therapeutic failure. Drug–food interactions and inappropriate off-label use also contribute significantly to serious adverse outcomes.

Patient-Related Factors:

Patient-specific characteristics play a critical role in the occurrence of SAEs. Age-related physiological changes in paediatric and geriatric populations affect drug absorption, metabolism, and excretion. Genetic polymorphisms influencing drug-metabolising enzymes may predispose individuals to severe reactions.

Comorbid conditions such as renal or hepatic impairment significantly increase susceptibility to SAEs. Pregnancy introduces additional ethical concerns, as drug exposure may affect both mother and foetus.

Healthcare System and Medication Errors:

System-level failures, including prescribing, dispensing, and administration errors, as well as inadequate monitoring, are preventable causes of SAEs. Poor communication among healthcare providers, a lack of standardised protocols, and insufficient patient education further increase the risk.

Ethically, preventable SAEs highlight systemic failures and reinforce the obligation to improve healthcare processes.

Pharmacovigilance Systems and Sae Reporting:

Pharmacovigilance encompasses activities aimed at detecting, assessing, and preventing adverse effects related to medicines. International coordination of pharmacovigilance activities is supported by the World Health Organization, which promotes global drug safety monitoring.

Most countries rely on spontaneous reporting systems for SAE detection. Regulatory agencies such as the Food and Drug Administration collect and analyse reports to identify safety signals and initiate regulatory action. While these systems are essential, their effectiveness depends heavily on ethical and proactive reporting by healthcare professionals and industry.

Pharmacovigilance is the cornerstone of drug safety monitoring. It encompasses activities related to the detection, assessment, understanding, and prevention of adverse drug effects.

Global pharmacovigilance efforts are supported by the World Health Organisation, which coordinates international drug safety monitoring through collaborative networks. At the national level, regulatory authorities collect and analyse SAE reports to identify safety signals.

The International Council for Harmonisation has developed standardised definitions and reporting requirements to harmonise SAE reporting across countries. In the United States, the Food and Drug Administration oversees post-marketing surveillance and regulatory action.

Despite established systems, spontaneous reporting remains largely voluntary, making ethical commitment from reporters essential for system effectiveness.

Ethical Principles Governing Sae Reporting:

- Ethical reporting of SAEs is rooted in fundamental principles of bioethics.
- Beneficence imposes a responsibility on healthcare professionals to act in the best interests of patients by preventing harm.
- Non-maleficence requires avoidance of actions that may cause injury, including failure to report serious risks.
- Respect for autonomy demands transparency so that patients can make informed decisions.
- Justice ensures equitable protection of all populations from drug-related harm.
- Together, these principles establish SAE reporting as a moral duty rather than a mere administrative task.

Ethical reporting of SAEs is grounded in core bioethical principles that guide healthcare practice and research.

Beneficence and Non-maleficence:

Beneficence requires actions that promote patient well-being, while non-maleficence emphasises avoidance of harm. Reporting SAEs enables early risk identification and the implementation of preventive measures, thereby fulfilling both principles.

Failure to report known or suspected SAEs constitutes ethical negligence, as it permits continued exposure to harm.

Respect for Patient Autonomy:

Patient autonomy depends on access to complete and accurate information. Ethical SAE reporting ensures that safety data inform prescribing decisions and patient consent processes. Without transparent reporting, patients are deprived of their right to make informed choices.

Justice and Equity:

Justice requires equitable protection of all patient populations. Underreporting of SAEs in vulnerable or underrepresented groups perpetuates healthcare inequities. Ethical pharmacovigilance ensures that drug safety data reflect real-world diversity.

Transparency and Professional Integrity:

Transparency in SAE reporting fosters trust among patients, healthcare professionals, and society. Professional integrity demands honesty, objectivity, and accountability in safety communication.

Ethical Responsibilities of Stakeholders:

Healthcare professionals bear primary responsibility for recognising and reporting SAEs encountered in practice. Researchers and clinical investigators must ensure rapid reporting during clinical trials, prioritising participant safety over scientific or commercial interests.

Pharmaceutical companies have an ethical obligation to monitor product safety throughout the drug lifecycle and to report SAEs without suppression or delay. Regulatory authorities are responsible for evaluating safety data objectively and taking timely action to protect public health.

Healthcare Professionals:

Healthcare professionals are ethically obligated to recognise, document, and report SAEs encountered in clinical practice. Reporting should be timely, accurate, and unbiased. Ethical practice prioritises patient safety over fear of blame or litigation.

Clinical Researchers and Investigators:

Investigators conducting clinical trials have a heightened ethical duty to protect participants. All SAEs must be promptly reported to sponsors, ethics committees, and regulatory authorities. Suppression or delay of SAE reporting violates research ethics and participant trust.

Pharmaceutical Industry:

Pharmaceutical companies are responsible for continuous safety monitoring throughout a product's lifecycle. Ethical responsibilities include transparent reporting, risk communication, and implementation of risk minimisation strategies. Commercial interests must never override patient safety.

Regulatory Authorities:

Regulatory agencies have an ethical responsibility to evaluate SAE data objectively and to take timely action. Delayed regulatory response can result in widespread harm, emphasising the importance of ethical governance.

Source Documentation:

Source Documentation of adverse events includes documentation in the medical records of:

- Event
- Date when it occurred
- Grade as determined by CTCAE (Common Terminology Criteria for Adverse Events)
- Expected or Unexpected
- Attribution as assigned by PI
- Date resolved
- The treatment the patient received was specifically related to events

Grading Adverse Events:

Minor: Transient or mild discomfort; no limitation in activity; no medical intervention/ therapy required

Moderate: Mild to moderate limitation in activity - some assistance may be needed; no or minimal medical intervention/ therapy required

Reporting Serious Events:

An investigator must promptly report to the sponsor and the IEC any adverse effect that may reasonably be regarded as caused by, or probably caused by, the drug. If the adverse effect is alarming, the investigator shall report it immediately. (*Rule 122DAC G.S.R. 63(E), 1 Feb 2013*)

Reporting Criteria:

- Routine Reporting
- Know which events can be reported at interim analysis or annual reviews, or as routine
- Expedited Reporting
- Know which events require reporting within the time frame
- Need to be familiar with the reporting requirements for your protocol
- Once again, be familiar with your protocol
- In some protocols, you will be responsible for providing data for the interim analysis (point where evaluate data) or for the annual review
- Need to know which events require immediate reporting

Regulations for SAE compensation:

- Drugs & Cosmetics (I Amendment) Rules, 2013 Gazette notification G.S.R. 53 (E), 30 Jan, 2013
- Drugs & Cosmetics (VI Amendment) Rules, 2014, Gazette notification G.S.R. 889 (E), 12 Dec, 2014
- Rule 122DAB: Compensation in case of injury/death during clinical trial

Compensation in Case of Injury or Death During Clinical Trial:

- In case of injury occurring to a participant
- Free medical management as long as required
- Till such time it is established that the injury is not related to the clinical trial, whichever is earlier

- If the injury / death is related to the clinical trial
- Entitled for financial compensation
- Over and above any expenses incurred on the medical management of the participant
- If no permanent injury, the quantum of compensation ... the nature of injury, loss of wages, transportation

Rule 122-DAB

Reasons for payment:

- Adverse effect of the investigational product
- Protocol violation, scientific misconduct, negligence
- Failure of the investigational product / use of placebo, in case the standard care was not provided
- Adverse effects due to concomitant medication excluding standard care
- Any clinical trial procedures involved in the study
- Injury to the child in-utero because of participation of parent in the clinical trial.

Rule 122- DAB

Formula for quantum of compensation (death):

Compensation for death = B x F x R / 99.37

Where B = Base amount (8 lakhs)

F = Factor depending on age

R = Risk factor (severity & seriousness, co-morbidities etc.

on a scale of 0.5 to 4)

actor (F) for calculating the amount of compensation

Age	Factors
1	2
16	228.54
17	227.49
18	226.38
19	225.22
20	224.00
21	222.71
22	221.37
23	219.95
24	218.47
25	216.91
26	215.28
27	213.57
28	211.79
29	209.92
30	207.98
31	205.95
32	203.85
33	201.66
34	199.40

Formula for quantum of compensation (other than death):

Permanent disability	(C x D x 90)/(100 x 100) D = Percentage of disability C = quantum of compensation payable in the event of death
SAE causing congenital anomaly Still birth & early death Correctable deformity &Permanent disability	Half of the amount as for death Medical management as long as required in addition to financial compensation
SAE causing life threatening disease & reversible SAE	2 x W x N W = Minimum wages for an unskilled worker in Delhi N = No. of days of hospitalization

Consequences of Improper Reporting:

- Research Privileges Revoked
- Suspend or cancel the trial
- Restrict the Sponsor from conducting any further clinical trials in the country
- Imprisonment for 1 year
- Fine not less than twice the amount of compensation
- Patient Safety

Challenges and Ethical Issues in Sae Reporting:

Major ethical challenges include underreporting, incomplete documentation, fear of legal consequences, and conflicts of interest. Inadequate pharmacovigilance infrastructure in low-resource settings further exacerbates inequities in drug safety monitoring.

Ethical concerns also arise when commercial interests influence the disclosure of safety information. Such practices undermine trust and violate professional and societal obligations.

One of the most persistent challenges in SAE reporting is underreporting. Contributing factors include lack of awareness, uncertainty regarding causality, time constraints, and fear of professional consequences.

Conflicts of interest pose serious ethical concerns, particularly in industry-sponsored research. Selective reporting or suppression of safety data undermines public trust and violates ethical norms.

Resource limitations and weak pharmacovigilance infrastructure in low- and middle-income countries further exacerbate global inequities in drug safety monitoring. Addressing these challenges requires systemic reforms, education, and ethical leadership.

Strategies to Strengthen Ethical Reporting:

Improving ethical SAE reporting requires education, simplified reporting mechanisms, and supportive institutional cultures. Integrating pharmacovigilance training into healthcare curricula and using electronic reporting tools can significantly enhance reporting rates.

International collaboration and transparent data sharing further strengthen global drug safety efforts.

Strengthening ethical reporting of serious adverse drug events is essential to enhance patient safety, improve drug regulation, and uphold professional integrity. Although pharmacovigilance systems exist worldwide, their effectiveness depends largely on the ethical commitment of healthcare professionals, researchers, pharmaceutical companies, and regulatory authorities. Multiple strategies have been proposed in the literature to improve both the quantity and quality of SAE reporting.

Education and Training in Pharmacovigilance:

One of the most effective strategies to improve ethical SAE reporting is education. Many healthcare professionals lack adequate training in recognising, documenting, and reporting adverse drug events. Integrating pharmacovigilance and ethics into undergraduate and postgraduate curricula for medicine, pharmacy, nursing, and allied health sciences can significantly improve reporting behaviour.

Continuing medical education (CME) programs and workshops focused on drug safety, ethical obligations, and reporting procedures help reinforce professional responsibility. Ethical education emphasises that reporting SAEs is not an act of blame but a contribution to collective learning and patient protection.

Simplification of Reporting Systems:

Complex and time-consuming reporting procedures are major barriers to SAE reporting. Simplifying reporting formats, minimising paperwork, and providing user-friendly electronic platforms can encourage the timely submission of reports. Online portals and mobile-based reporting applications reduce practical obstacles and support real-time reporting.

Ethically, simplifying systems respects the constraints faced by busy healthcare professionals while promoting responsible behaviour. User-centred design of reporting tools improves accuracy and completeness of data, enhancing overall pharmacovigilance outcomes.

Promotion of a Non-Punitive Reporting Culture:

Fear of legal action, professional criticism, or institutional punishment often discourages reporting of serious adverse drug events. Establishing a non-punitive and blame-free culture is critical to ethical reporting. Healthcare institutions should emphasise learning and system improvement rather than individual fault.

Such a culture aligns with ethical principles of beneficence and justice by encouraging transparency and collective responsibility. When healthcare professionals feel supported rather than threatened, reporting rates and data quality improve significantly.

Strengthening Institutional and Organisational Support:

Hospitals and healthcare organisations play a vital role in promoting ethical SAE reporting. Establishing pharmacovigilance committees, appointing trained drug safety officers, and providing clear reporting guidelines can strengthen institutional accountability.

Regular feedback to reporters regarding the outcomes of submitted SAE reports reinforces the value of reporting and sustains ethical motivation. Organisational leadership must actively support safety initiatives to embed ethical pharmacovigilance into routine clinical practice.

Role of Regulatory Frameworks and Policies:

Strong regulatory frameworks are essential for ensuring ethical reporting of SAEs. Clear legal requirements for reporting, defined timelines, and standardised procedures promote consistency and accountability. Regulatory authorities must balance enforcement with education to avoid discouraging voluntary reporting.

Ethically sound regulations protect public health while respecting professional autonomy. Transparent communication of regulatory decisions and safety alerts further strengthens trust in the healthcare system.

International Collaboration and Data Sharing:

Drug safety is a global concern, as medicines are marketed and used across national boundaries. International collaboration and sharing of SAE data enhance early signal detection and risk assessment. Collaborative networks coordinated by the World Health Organisation facilitate global pharmacovigilance and ethical exchange of safety information.

Ethical data sharing ensures that knowledge gained from one population benefits others, promoting global justice and equity in healthcare.

Future Perspectives:

The future of serious adverse drug event reporting lies at the intersection of technological innovation, ethical governance, and patient-centred care. Emerging tools and evolving ethical frameworks offer opportunities to enhance drug safety while presenting new challenges that must be carefully addressed.

Emerging technologies such as electronic health records, real-world evidence, and artificial intelligence offer promising tools for early detection of serious adverse drug events. Ethical implementation of these technologies must ensure patient privacy, data security, and equitable access.

Digital Health and Electronic Reporting Systems:

The widespread adoption of electronic health records (EHRs) has created new opportunities for automated detection and reporting of SAEs. Integration of pharmacovigilance modules within EHR systems allows real-time identification of potential adverse events, reducing reliance on voluntary reporting alone.

From an ethical perspective, digital reporting systems can improve the completeness and timeliness of data while minimising the reporting burden. However, safeguards must be in place to protect patient confidentiality and data security.

Use of Artificial Intelligence and Big Data:

Artificial intelligence (AI) and machine learning algorithms are increasingly being explored for pharmacovigilance applications. These technologies can analyse large datasets from clinical records, registries, and spontaneous reporting systems to identify safety signals earlier than traditional methods.

While AI offers significant potential, ethical concerns include algorithmic transparency, the risk of bias, and accountability for decision-making. Ethical implementation requires human oversight, model validation, and clear accountability for regulatory actions based on AI-generated signals.

Patient-Centred and Consumer Reporting:

The future of SAE reporting increasingly recognises the role of patients and consumers. Patient-reported outcomes and direct reporting of adverse events provide valuable real-world insights into drug safety. Empowering patients to report SAEs enhances autonomy and inclusiveness.

Ethically, patient involvement democratizes pharmacovigilance and ensures that safety systems reflect lived experiences. Education and accessible reporting tools are essential to support meaningful patient participation.

Ethical Governance and Transparency:

As pharmacovigilance systems evolve, ethical governance will remain central. Transparent disclosure of safety data, open communication of risks, and clear explanation of regulatory decisions are essential for maintaining public trust.

Future ethical frameworks must address conflicts of interest, ensure independence of regulatory authorities, and promote accountability across all stakeholders. Ethical leadership will be crucial in balancing innovation with patient protection.

Global Equity and Capacity Building:

Strengthening pharmacovigilance capacity in low- and middle-income countries is a key future priority. Global equity requires investment in infrastructure, training, and regulatory support to ensure that all populations benefit equally from drug safety monitoring.

Ethically, addressing global disparities in SAE reporting reflects principles of justice and solidarity. International partnerships and funding initiatives play a vital role in building sustainable pharmacovigilance systems worldwide.

Conclusion:

Serious adverse drug events represent one of the most significant challenges in modern pharmacotherapy, with profound implications for patient safety, public health, and healthcare systems worldwide. Despite advances in drug development and regulatory science, no medicinal product is entirely devoid of risk. The occurrence of serious adverse events underscores the necessity of continuous monitoring throughout a drug's lifecycle and highlights the critical role of ethical reporting in safeguarding patients.

This work has emphasised that serious adverse drug events are not merely clinical occurrences but ethical concerns that demand transparency, accountability, and professional integrity. Ethical reporting of SAEs enables early detection of safety signals, facilitates evidence-based regulatory decisions, and prevents the recurrence of avoidable harm. The principles of beneficence, non-maleficence, respect for autonomy, and justice provide the moral foundation for pharmacovigilance activities and reinforce the reporting of adverse events as a professional obligation rather than an optional administrative task.

The responsibilities associated with SAE reporting are shared among multiple stakeholders, including healthcare professionals, researchers, pharmaceutical manufacturers, and regulatory authorities. Each plays a vital role in ensuring that safety information is accurately identified, promptly communicated, and appropriately acted upon. Failures in ethical reporting—whether due to underreporting, conflicts of interest, or system limitations—can result in widespread harm and erosion of public trust in medicines and healthcare institutions.

While existing pharmacovigilance systems have significantly improved drug safety monitoring, persistent challenges remain. Underreporting, inadequate infrastructure, fear of blame, and global disparities in reporting capacity continue to limit the effectiveness of SAE surveillance. Addressing these challenges requires sustained education, supportive reporting environments, strong regulatory frameworks, and ethical leadership at institutional, national, and international levels.

Looking ahead, emerging technologies such as electronic health records, real-world evidence, artificial intelligence, and patient-centred reporting offer promising opportunities to enhance the detection and management of serious adverse drug events. However, the ethical implementation of these innovations must prioritise patient privacy, transparency, and equitable access to ensure that technological progress translates into meaningful improvements in drug safety.

In conclusion, ethical reporting of serious adverse drug events is fundamental to responsible healthcare practice and effective pharmacovigilance. Strengthening ethical awareness, fostering a culture of transparency, and reinforcing shared responsibility among all stakeholders are essential to minimising drug-related harm. Through continuous commitment to ethical reporting, healthcare systems can transform adverse events into valuable learning opportunities, ultimately ensuring safer and more effective use of medicines for all populations.

References:

1. National ethical guidelines for biomedical and health research involving human participants

2. New Drugs and Clinical Trials Rules 2019 G.S.R. 227(E) Central Drugs Standard Control Organisation, Directorate General of Health Services, Ministry of Health & Family Welfare, Government of India

3. Central Drugs Standard Control Organisation (CDSCO) User Manual for SAE reporting (Serious Adverse Event) on the SUGAM portal .

Chapter 12

Data Protection and Privacy in Research-Ethics

Dr. Krishnendu Mukhopadhyay
Professor
EHE-SRFPH, SRIHER
E-Mail: krishnendu@sriramachandra.edu.in

Objectives:

Principally, all the four fundamental ethical principles, e.g., autonomy, beneficence, non-maleficence, and justice are essential inclusions in implementing research ethics. However, the special attentions that are required to fulfil the objectives are –

- To maintain the sustainable research ethics in terms of data protection and privacy of the recruited study participants with fullest accountability, transparency and trust
- To safeguard participants personal data aligned to the respective research study and are within the standard protocol, guidelines and compliance measures.

In addition, protection of ultrasensitive human and animal data need stringent adherence to comply ethical guidelines addressing privacy, integrity and safety norms of the research activities.

Keywords:

Data Protection, Data Privacy, Research Ethics, Anonymisation, Policy

Introduction:

It's a fact that the protection and maintaining personal data-privacy demand people's right. Poor **data protection and privacy** in research may be harmful to participants by breaching public trust that may lead to legal complexities. It may also damage scientific integrity which is crucial in research ethics. Institutions handling public data should be safeguarded cautiously while collecting, processing, analysing or publishing irrespective of concerns and contexts. Here the research work included with humans or animals secures data protection.

Data protection should safeguard subjects' dignity, rights, and/or freedoms in the processing of personal data. It is the national and/or international directives that legitimise the scopes and conditions of personal data processing. Project funding agencies also seek evidence-based assurance of data protection to ensure time-bound research activities proceed smoothly. It is imperative to note that the data protection protocol also encourages researchers to inform participants of the study results. This protective mechanism should be supported with a stringent follow-up process by the research organisations or institutes.

On the other hand, **data privacy** is a set of guidelines for collecting or handling data based on its sensitivity and importance. Data privacy is very important in the context of the United Nations Sustainable Development Goals (SDGs), too. Preserving data integrity endorses social justice (SDG 16) that backs sustainable development. Data privacy should be the primary responsibility that ensures participants' inclusion is protected in research studies. It's not the selection of an individual or so-called study subject that matters only, but together with compliance and objective protocols, overall procedures starting from subject recruitment till data collection and analysis should be under privacy guidelines. None other than the study-relevant information from the subjects is approved by the allied research ethics board or committee. In addition, the technical aspects like the data management system with whatever advancements should be primarily ensured with data quality.

Importance of Data Protection:

Steps endorse data protection by ensuring the legitimate privacy, accessibility, and integrity of sensitive data. However, the terms data protection and data security, though used interchangeably, focus on technical security by preventing unauthorised intervention in the integrated process of ensuring data confidentiality, data compliance and data management.

Its principles help in protecting data to such an extent that it makes it available as and when the circumstances demand it. Operational and developmental data backup or recovery processes of data protection are also included in the integrated data management system.

Considering research ethics in India, data protection needs stringent confidentiality, spontaneity in informed consent, and complied data validity as per the Indian Council of Medical Research (ICMR) guidelines. Governance in the use of data protection also follows the Digital Personal Data Protection

(DPDP) Act, 2023 (Govt. of India) that aims to balance individual privacy.

ICMR Guidelines on Data Protection & Privacy in research ethics:

In the ICMR guidelines (2017 & 2023 AI updates), stringent mandate has been created and circulated on data protection and privacy in biomedical research where special emphases have been highlighted upon informed consent, confidentiality, and participant safety. Anonymization, data storage security up to 5 years, and ethical oversight for data usages have been considered as very important segments with special emphasis in artificial intelligence and bio-banking.

Key Principles are:

- **Informed Consent**: It is embedded in the principles of the Nuremberg Code, the Declaration of Helsinki and the Belmont Report. Informed consent is an essential requirement prior to any research involving human subjects. Participants must be informed about the data collected, its purpose, confidentiality measures, and their right to withdraw.
- **Confidentiality & Privacy:** These are ethical and legitimate obligations of researchers to use personal data securely and prevent leaks, especially in digital formats.
- **Data Minimisation & Anonymisation**: In research ethics, data minimisation is the practice of collecting, storing, and utilising only the data necessary to meet study objectives. It protects participant privacy, reduces the risk of data breaches, and ensures compliance with national and international regulations. On the other hand, data anonymisation is a key

component of the qualitative research process, involving the removal or alteration of personal identifiers to protect participants' privacy.

- **Security Measures**: It prioritises participant privacy through technical, physical, and administrative safeguards. Security measures ensure compliance with robust data security strategies, including disaster recovery plans and Information Technology (IT) breach safeguards.
- **Retention Period**: In India, ethical research data, especially from clinical trials, must generally be retained for a minimum of 5 years after study completion, though certain health records may require longer retention. For biomedical research, records must be maintained for at least 3 years and for clinical trials, 5 years after the completion of the study.
- **AI & Big Data Regulations (2023):** Guidelines for AI in healthcare emphasise data privacy, bias minimisation, trustworthiness, and transparency. Digital Personal Data Protection Act (DPDP Act) 2023 in August 2023. This act provides the foundational legal framework for data privacy, impacting how AI models are trained, how big data is managed, and the ethical documentation required for research.
- **Data Sharing and Transfer:** A Data Sharing Agreement (DSA) is a legally binding contract between two or more parties that outlines the terms and conditions for data sharing. In collaborative research, material transfer agreements (MTAs) and data sharing agreements are mandatory to ensure protection

Digital Personal Data Protection (DPDP) Rule, 2025 (Govt. of India):

The Government of India notified the Digital Personal Data Protection Rules, 2025, on November 13, 2025, which enforced the Digital Personal Data Protection Act, 2023 (DPDP Act). It focuses on citizen data rights, consent mechanisms, and data fiduciary obligations. The DPDP Rules 2025 made India's data protection law fully operational by translating the DPDP Act into enforceable procedures.

Key Features of the DPDP Rules, 2025

- **Consent & Notice:** As per India's DPDP Rules, 2025, consent must be free, specific, informed, unconditional, and unambiguous, and must be obtained through clear affirmative action. Data Fiduciaries must provide clear, simple, and itemised notices for exploring data purposes. Withdrawing consent must be as easy as giving it, with an 18-month phased compliance period.
- **Data Protection Board of India:** It's a 4–member digital board, established for complaint filing and grievance redressal via a portal/app. Four members will be able to file complaints online and track their cases through a dedicated portal and mobile application. This digital platform enables faster decision-making and simplifies grievance redressal. Provisions of appeals against the Board's decisions may be heard by the Appellate Tribunal, TDSAT.
- **Children's Data:** DPDP Rules set very stringent child-data safeguards, but their impact are depended upon the way of the implementation by the schools & parents. Verifiable parental/guardian consent is mandatory before processing, with exceptions for essential services.

- **Breach Notification:** From ransomware attacks and phishing-driven intrusions to misconfigured cloud servers and insider threats, breaches occur across industries, jurisdictions, and platforms. Recognising this risk, the DPDP Act, 2023 and the DPDP Rules, 2025 introduce one of India's most comprehensive and enforceable breach notification regimes, centred on Rule 7. Under this, the organisations must immediately notify affected individuals and the Board of any breaches, followed by a detailed report within 72 hours.
- **Security & Retention**: Data retention is where good intentions in data protection often succeed or fail. It is to be noted that the retention does not merely mean to keep data forever with some expected outcomes, but to be deliberate by assuring a genuine need for a lawful purpose. The rest can be deleted in a way that allows explanation, repetition, and auditing.
- **Rights of Data Principals**: Data Principals (individuals) have strengthened rights to access, correct, erase, and object to the processing of their data, with data fiduciaries required to respond within 90 days. Key rights include withdrawing consent, nominating representatives, and seeking grievance redressal.
- **Significant Data Fiduciaries (SDFs):** These are entities designated by the Indian government under the DPDP Act 2023 and 2025 Rules based on risk factors like data volume, sensitivity, and national security impact. They face higher compliance, including mandatory Data Protection Impact Assessments (DPIA), annual audits, appointing an India-based Data Protection Officer (DPO), and strict algorithmic, cross-border data transfer, and reporting obligations.

Importance of Data Privacy:

Data privacy safeguards legal compliances by paying respect to the autonomy and trust of the study subjects which help reducing the risk of illegal intervention. That means data privacy in research-ethics secures personal data from any unauthorized access to maintain confidentiality and upholding informed consent. Data protection is an important tool to preserve personal health information (PHI) and personally identifiable information (PII) and retains social security as a whole.

While discussing research ethics, researchers must minimize harm, prevent misuse, and respect autonomy. However in research data protection and privacy the following considerations are must -

- Focussed ethical principles
- Understanding Belmont report
- Organizing functional research ethics board
- Respecting the subjects either on accepting or rejecting informed consent
- Ascertaining maximum benefits and minimum risks of the subjects recruited
- Proper screening of questionnaire to avoid unnecessary data

The Indian Council of Medical Research emphasizes that ethics committees (ECs) are responsible for overseeing privacy measures in research projects.

While considering digital health research and ethics, data privacy for industrial system is equally important. Adequate ethics coverage may sensitize complex entities of the industrial research paradigm, may it be their administrative core or the workers personal data, to maintain stringent protection and privacy addressing industrial sector. Data collection, third-party sharing, data storage etc. must oblige legitimate consideration and ethical issues that are reflected in commercial settings. In fact some of the domains are not under preview of legal compliance, but remain in the ethical responsibility while addressing research ethics. One prime example in this domain may include acquiring consent from the participants or from specific authorities.

Data Protection vs Data Privacy:

Both, data protection and data privacy in research-ethics are inevitable domains and are very close to each other while understanding the notes in the context of ethical research. Data updates in terms of best community or clinical research protection and privacy of public data should be secured from any possible cyberattacks and data breaches.

When comparing data protection and data privacy, the core area of the individual parameter needs to be understood clearly. Data protection is allowed to all forms of data whether it is personal or organizational. It is primarily based upon available data and its safe custody from the risks of unauthorized access or harm. It accomplishes the policy and procedure guidelines. It also ensures data integrity and availability by safeguarding data from unauthorized access, damage or hijack. In nutshell, the general taglines are: "How the data gets protected" & "What are the required Safety measures" embedded with. Here, the focus should be to prevent data breaching. Mitigating data leaking, anonymization and pseudonymization are other forms of responsible acts of data protection.

But, on the other hand, data privacy is concerned with the individual's control over their personal information. However, here the taglines are: Why is Data Privacy important" and "What are the precautionary measure" adopted to sustain data privacy. In this case, the focus would be on autonomy, informed consent, and confidentiality of the study participants. In data privacy, participants' wishes would have prime importance, especially in having the right to the detailed information of the data collected from them and at any time they can revoke the consent. Addressing GDPR or IRB regulations is another core of data privacy.

Sensitive Data in the Contexts of Research Ethics:

Sensitive data in the context of research ethics requires utmost protection and privacy of the information collected from the study participants. Violation of the protocol may harm privacy of the participants and is a direct breach of contract. Sensitive data includes genetic data, health data, issues related to illegal activities or sexual behaviour, etc.

Stringent protocols and standards should be maintained to protect the data collected from sensitive or at-risk populations. It may span any age group within the target population of the study. As mentioned, sensitive data in research ethics requires strict confidentiality. In parallel, legal and ethical standards need to be maintained very strictly for vulnerable population too. In some cases, some geopolitical/religious data are also notified as sensitive data where no direct personal connection is observed. Anonymising personal data or with proper informed consent, one can ensure data preservation for long-term access. However, ethical handling suggests data optimization to ensure smooth chain of custody from collecting informed consent through data dissemination.

Conducting research with vulnerable populations (ex: children, political critics, prisoners, sex workers etc.) needs special attention of data protection and privacy as disclosing their identification may cause significant harm to them. In this case, extra safeguards can help data confidentiality by following up optimized data collection, limited data access and stringent data storage management. For collaborative research, researchers should ensure data privacy that meets any policy requirements related to collaborations based on funding-resource, institutional affiliation and citizenship of the individuals.

For ultrasensitive data protection, maintenance of rigorous protocols is must for vulnerable population data. However, special care is adopted for these ultra-cases to avoid unauthorized access, breach, or disclosure. In addition, data security is treated as a fundamental human right rather than just a legal compliance requirement.

In addition, the 7 core rules of the General Data Protection Regulation (GDPR, European Union) such as Lawfulness, Fairness & Transparency; Purpose Limitation; Data Minimisation; Accuracy; Storage Limitation; Integrity & Confidentiality; and Accountability are also taken into account while handling of personal data **(Figure – 1).**

Data Security in Research Ethics:

Data security is another important segment in research ethics where data protection and privacy are warranted. Technological advancements, cost-benefit analysis and robust procedural data management ensures data incubation and any chance of data breaching from any angle. To combat data security breach from any potential risks personal data should be de-identified, as and when required, with affirmative aggregation pseudonymization, or masking. Where appropriate, The United Nations Sustainable Development Group should be alert to ensure data security process that has been de-identified/masked by third party data providers.

In India, data security in research ethics is primarily guided by the Digital Personal Data Protection Act (DPDPA), 2023. Specific use of research data should comply with the Information Technology Act 2000, too.

In Indian research ethics, the data security framework has been considered as a very important landscape that ensures check and balance between the rapid digitization of data and the fundamental right to privacy recognized by the Supreme Court in 2017. The data security framework is very much embedded in ethical principles, guidelines, legal statutes, and sectoral policies that emphasize informed consent, data minimization, and stringent security measures **(Table – 1).**

Data Retention and Data Minimization:

Data retention and security in Indian research are governed by the Digital Personal Data Protection Act (DPDPA) 2023 and ICMR guidelines. In this concern, special emphasis is given on data minimization, confidentiality and informed consent of the participants. Important parameters involved in data retention and security in India includes DPDPA 2023 compliance, ICMR guidelines, Data security measures, Data custodianship, and rights of data subjects. DPDPA 2023 directs data deletion once the purpose of the data is fulfilled or when the participants withdraw their participatory consents. ICMR suggests allied ethics committee to look after the matter related to secured data retention and research integrity. Data security measures are subdivided by three important parameters, namely: a. Physical Storage, b. Electronic Storage and c. Anonymization. Data custodianship is ensured with data retention as per legitimate time limit is prescribed. Study participants are also dignified by being empowered to have every right to delete their personal data from the research study, on request.

To retain data in research ethics intact, specific objectives and hypotheses of the study may help minimise data burden to reach the research goal. Actually, the provision of data retention and collection starts from the objectives and expected outcomes of the research study. A feasible, innovative, and concise strategy limits the data-retention burden. In addition, proper implementation of monitoring protocol with stringent guidelines may form the basis of specific data collection and retention in ethical research. Storing potentially sensitive data should always be handled with care and sensitivity, given the associated risks, harms, and benefits. Deletion of any public research data should only be permitted as per the standard legitimate protocol that maintains data sensitivity.

In India, data retention related to research ethics ensures data security, data anonymisation, and data storage for 3 to 5 years after the completion of the study, with audits and reproducibility compliance. In addition, researchers must follow the institutional policies that may require three copies, two different media, and one off-site rule.

Data Quality:

In research ethics, data quality must be ensured through rigorous accuracy, validity, and integrity to produce sound scientific data. This is in accordance with ICMR mandates to ensure stringent guidelines against data falsification or plagiarism. Obviously, participants' data protection and privacy are key components of the institutional oversight committees, safeguarded by required accountability and transparency. All data-related activities should be designed, carried out, reported, and documented with an adequate level of quality and transparency. More specifically, data should be validated for accuracy, relevance, sufficiency, integrity, completeness, usability, validity, and coherence, and kept up to date.

In the context of risks, data quality needs to be preserved carefully so that low and high-quality data are distinctly separated and are treated meticulously.

In recent years, quality research ethics data in the context of documentation and privacy have shown tremendous growth in India. Considering rapid expansion and success in clinical trials, Indian researchers encourage seriousness very much upon the quality data and screen uneven and misconducted research data separately for adequate actions through legal enforcement measures.

Processing personal data in research:

Data processing is a very important concern in research ethics. It has a wide spectrum of custodians involved in various steps of data processing, such as handling, analysing, and storing data, all while maintaining proper privacy and confidentiality. The main areas of data processing include: editing, coding, classification, tabulation and diagram. The process starts from its raw form and converts it into readable texts with technological support and individual interpretations. Normally, there are six stages of data processing, namely – collection, preparation, input, processing, output and reporting. Data having common characteristics are classified before further subdivisions.

Personal data processing in research are adhered with stringent data protection principles of the investigating agency or institute. Personal data processing must be accompanied with core requirements of the study that includes obtaining explicit, informed, and revocable consent, enforcing data minimization, ensuring secure storage/encryption, and anonymizing data to prevent identification.

Legal basis for processing personal data may be under two categories of personal data: 'non-sensitive' and 'sensitive' personal data. This distinction is important because processing sensitive personal data is prohibited unless stringent conditions are met **(Figure -2).** Common parameters of personal data processing are –

- Consent
- Contractual necessity
- Legal obligation
- Vital interests and
- Legitimate interests

It is to be noted that the GDPR is the European Union's comprehensive data privacy law, effective since May 25, 2018, that mandates strict rules on collecting, storing, and processing personal data. Navigating GDPR compliance involves understanding consent intricacies, choosing appropriate lawful bases, and respecting individuals' rights.

Legal frameworks and consent, Data minimisation and purpose limitation, Transparency and fair processing, Data security and transcription, Cross-border data transfer, Data retention and deletion and Third-party processors and contracts are different stages of collecting and processing personal data **(Figure 3).**

The DPDP Rules, 2025, enforced strict guidelines on the data processing in research that include 72-hour breach reporting, 90-day grievance redressal, mandatory parental consent for children and a strict auditing system for significant data fiduciaries. Any entity processing personal data within India, or outside India in connection with offering goods or services to data principals in India, may transfer personal data to a foreign state or persons/entities under its control only if it complies with restrictions imposed by the Indian Government on the transfer of such data.

The Indian Government has designated Significant Data Fiduciaries (SDFs) to address the high risks associated with processed data under the DPDP Act 2023. Nowadays, data processing using artificial intelligence (AI) has become another challenge in the context of data protection, processing and privacy, and these need to be addressed under protection compliance. They face many complex, legitimate challenges in the domains of Data Protection Officers (DPOs), Data Protection Impact Assessments (DPIAs), and audits.

Images depicting data processing in research ethics highlight the responsible handling of information through icons and scenes representing privacy, security, and compliance. Common visuals include biometric pads, encrypted databases, informed consent forms, and collaborative teams that ensure fairness and transparency, frequently utilising blue gradients, linear, and schematic styles to convey trust and integrity.

Data Management Plan:

A Data Management Plan (DMP) is a formal document detailing how research data is handled, stored, secured, and shared, ensuring compliance with ethical standards and privacy regulations like GDPR. It is a document, written in advance of a project, which is used to capture and communicate information about -

- What data will be collected or created
- How it will be documented and described
- Where the data will be stored and responsibility for data security
- Which data will be shared and/or preserved
- How it will be shared and with whom

DMP addresses informed consent, data anonymization, secure storage, and retention policies to protect participants, often required by funders for FAIR data management (Findable, Accessible, Interoperable, and Reusable).

In fact, the DMP is a roadmap for collecting, storing, documenting, and sharing research data throughout a project. It ensures:

- Secure and ethically handled
- Well-documented, organised, and responsibly planned
- Preserved for long-term access

- Accessible, shareable, and reusable, when appropriate

The whole process encourages thinking about the life of the collected data after the end of the project. It will also help to -

- Anticipate and prepare for problems
- Mitigate against the risk of losing data or duplicating effort
- Define and communicate a consistent approach
- Safeguard the reliability, accuracy, safety and completeness of data

When conducting research, researchers actively and systematically manage data protection and information security. Data must be processed for lawful purposes and only to the extent necessary for carrying out the research.

The principles of data protection must be addressed while taking research datasets available to the academic community or for publications. Necessary agreements pertaining to the processing of personal data must be concluded with partners or subcontractors. However, researcher must inform the study participants in a very transparent manner by considering-

- Research content
- Processing of personal data
- Study subjects' rights related to the processing of personal data

Principal investigators must address the competency of the subordinates who practices in processing personal data before the commencement. They must specify the responsibilities and duties of processing personal data included in research materials based on the roles of the staff (coordinator, contact person or processor). They are also responsible for ensuring that the projects comply with data protection legislation and the data protection principles as are governed by the national standards and protocols.

Conclusion:

Data protection and privacy in research ethics needs mutual trust between researchers and participants. It requires careful planning, utmost transparency, and stringent compliance that maintain required compliance measures to safeguard personal information of the study participants. In recent years, with all-around technological advancements, research datasets are very much dependent upon digital form which needs to be protected with extra care. It has to be ensured that participant rights and the integrity are protected with evidential standardized proofs in the context of data protection and privacy.

References:

1. Jacqlyn L Yourell, Kelsey L McAlister, Clare C Beatty, Jennifer L Huberty; Exploring Ethics: Understanding the Role of Privacy Policies and Institutional Review Boards in Digital Health Companies; Journal of Medical Internet Research; 2025 May 16;27:e70711. doi: 10.2196/70711

2. Ethical Guidelines for Bio-Medical Research on Human Participants, Indian Council of Medical Research, 2006

3. Guidance on writing a Data Management Plan (DMP), University of Dundee, Updated on 16 October 2024

Annexure 1

Table 1: Data Security Framework in Indian Research Ethics

Ethical Component	**Requirements and Best Practices in India**	**Relevant Guidelines/ Laws**
Informed Consent	Voluntary, written, and informed consent must clearly explain data usage, storage, and sharing. Data Principals have the right to withdraw consent at any time.	ICMR Guidelines 2017; DPDPA 2023
Data Minimization	Only data necessary for the specific research objective should be collected, used, and retained.	DPDPA 2023
Confidentiality	Identifiable information (names, photos, addresses) must be kept confidential and not disclosed to unauthorized individuals.	ICMR Guidelines 2017; IT Act 2000

Ethical Component	Requirements and Best Practices in India	Relevant Guidelines/ Laws
Anonymization	Data must be anonymized or pseudonymized immediately after collection to prevent participant identification.	ICMR Guidelines 2017; DPDPA 2023
Secure Storage	Digital data must be encrypted, and physical records must be locked securely. Access must be restricted to authorized personnel (role-based access).	DPDPA 2023; IT Rules 2011
Data Retention	Research records should be maintained for a specific period (3 years for health, 5 years for clinical trials) after study completion, then destroyed securely.	ICMR Policy on RIPE; DPDPA 2023
Data Sharing	Data sharing with third parties or international partners requires valid, contractual agreements (MoU/MTA) ensuring equivalent protection.	ICMR Guidelines 2017; DPDPA 2023

Ethical Component	Requirements and Best Practices in India	Relevant Guidelines/ Laws
Breach Management	Data fiduciaries must notify the Data Protection Board of India and affected individuals in case of a data breach.	DPDPA 2023; CERT-In Directions
Research Misconduct	Fabrication, falsification, or plagiarism of data is prohibited. Data must be verifiable.	ICMR Policy on RIPE

Source: Ethical Guidelines for Bio-Medical Research on Human Participants, ICMR, 2006

Annexure 2

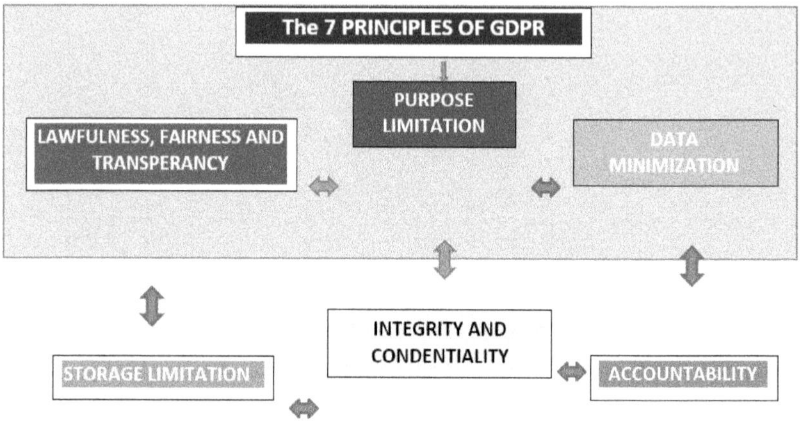

Figure 1: The Principles of GDPR

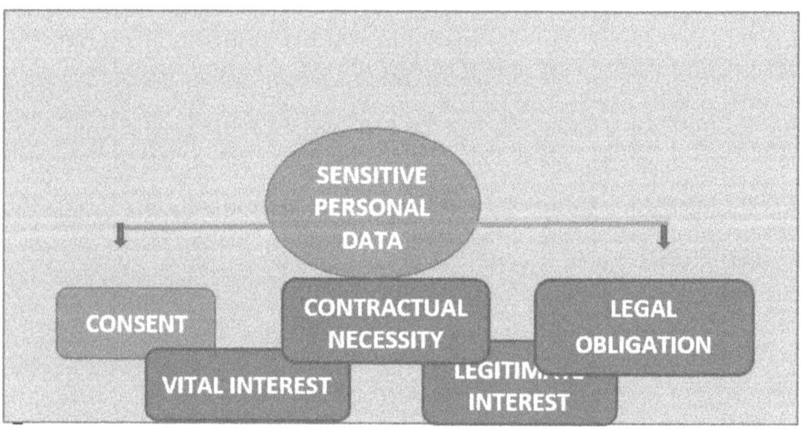

figure 2: Compliance of processing personal data

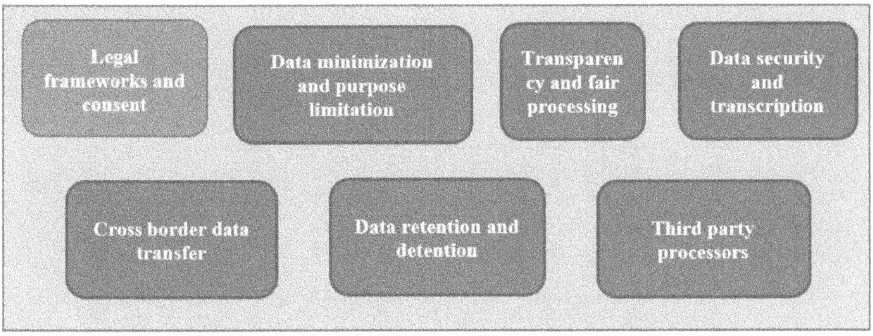

Figure 3: Collection and processing of personal data

Synopsis

Fundamentals of Research and Good Clinical Practice is a structured and comprehensive resource designed to equip learners and professionals with the essential knowledge and skills required for ethical and effective research conduct. Developed in accordance with UGC and ICMR standards, the book emphasizes the integration of scientific methodology with ethical responsibility.

The book covers key areas including research design, clinical trial processes, regulatory requirements, ethical review mechanisms, informed consent, data management, and publication ethics. Each chapter is authored by experienced ethics committee members and domain experts, ensuring both academic depth and practical relevance.

Special focus is given to Good Clinical Practice (GCP) guidelines, participant rights and safety, and maintaining integrity in research and publication. Through clear explanations and real-world perspectives, the book aims to foster a culture of ethical awareness and scientific accountability.

This text is particularly valuable for undergraduate and postgraduate students, early-career researchers, clinicians, and faculty members involved in research and academic activities. It serves not only as a learning resource but also as a reference guide for conducting responsible, transparent, and high-quality research.

www.ingramcontent.com/pod-product-compliance
Lightning Source LLC
LaVergne TN
LVHW050927210926
848482LV00013B/560
9798903629367